Psych
Your Diet

A DAILY DOSE

Volume 2

Psych Yourself to

STICK TO IT

Psych Your Diet

A DAILY DOSE

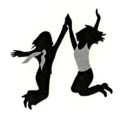

Volume 2
Psych Yourself to
STICK TO IT

Kenneth Schwarz PhD
Julie North Schwarz

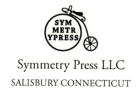

Symmetry Press LLC
SALISBURY CONNECTICUT

Publisher's Cataloging-In-Publication Data
(Prepared by The Donohue Group, Inc.)

Schwarz, Kenneth.
   Psych your diet. Volume 2, Psych yourself to stick to it : a daily dose / Kenneth Schwarz, Julie North Schwarz.
      p. ; cm.
   Issued also as an eBook.
   ISBN: 978-0-9774777-5-3
      1. Weight loss--Psychological aspects.   2. Reducing diets--Psychological aspects.   I. Ellyn, Julie.   II. Title.   III. Title: Psych yourself to stick to it

RM222.2 .S39 2010 v.1
613.2/5   2010935007

Cover illustration by Paula North
Book Design by DesignForBooks.com

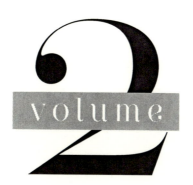

volume 2

Psych Your Diet:
A Daily Dose Volume 2.

Introduction

TO THE SERIES

Psych Your Diet

A DAILY DOSE

If you are having trouble sticking to a weight-loss plan, this is a good place to get help.

And remember…

Successful dieting is mostly psychological. The psychological part may even count as much as 95%. The psychological part is about psyching yourself to

START

STICK TO IT

KEEP IT OFF

If DIET and EXERCISE make up only 5%, you won't have what you need in order to lose weight.

For the other 95%, you need to pay attention to the psychological side of dieting and weight loss. That's when losing weight becomes a lot easier for you.

And that's what this series is all about.

Put This Book to Work for You

Self-help isn't really self-help unless someone else is also helping you. We'd like to be that someone.

If you want to solve a difficult weight problem, you need to be able to stick to your resolve.

This book is designed so you can read one piece at a time, one a day. You can think of it as a dose of daily knowhow, encouragement, and inspiration. Savor each idea, think about its implications, compare it with what you know, and try it out.

Each selection has its place on the psychological side of dieting and weight loss. You may find yourself coming back to some of the readings over and over again. Concepts that are not relevant at one time can become absolutely essential later on.

Go ahead and take each daily dose. Psych yourself as you go, every day.

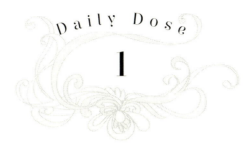

I totally reject the idea that some sort of underlying psychology is at work here.

That's your prerogative, of course.

> If you stay on a diet, you'll lose the weight. If you don't, you won't.

Sounds right.

> The rest is all mumbo-jumbo.

You can certainly look at it that way.

> I mean, I know why I don't lose weight. It's because I can't even stick to my diet.

Good point.

> It's pretty clear-cut, don't you see?

I do.

> All I need to do is actually stick to the diet, and I'll be thin. It's

straightforward, despite all your theories.

Yes.

I'll just stick to it this time

How will you be able to do that?

I have no idea.

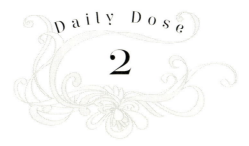

Daily Dose

2

marriage has its comings and goings, its ins and outs, ups and downs. So does a friendship, a career path, a family, as well as every day of life. A diet does too.

Sticking with it doesn't mean a smooth ride, an easy ride, an uncomplicated ride. But sticking with a diet is a lot of times every bit as important as sticking with all the other essentials of life.

Sticking with a diet is important not because it's a whim—to get thinner than your best friend. It isn't important because everyone is on one diet or another. It isn't important in order to be model-thin, to fit into a tiny size 2.

Sticking with a diet is important only when a woman's life, her comfort and happiness, are being compromised by her weight. It is only when an eating problem troubles her, and gets in her way, that it becomes so important to solve.

Many women suffer because they use eating to supply things they are not getting—meaningful things, things they need. This is when a diet becomes a make or break issue.

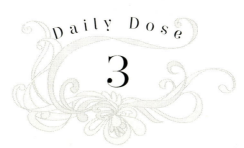

Daily Dose

3

Whatever food plan you choose, the real work of losing weight goes on inside. The work is thoughtful, it's questioning. It's a matter of feeling; it's a matter of time; it's a matter of increasing awareness; it's a matter of opening up your heart to yourself.

The real work is very different from the hustle and bustle of the diet itself, with weighing and planning and preparing and measuring and counting. The real work of dieting isn't the noisy part, it's the quiet part.

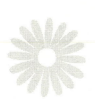

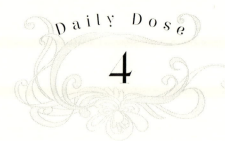

Daily Dose

4

Do you let things wreck your diet? . . . habits and husbands and weather and kids and the first of May and December 31st and weekends and headaches and colds and gray winters and hot summers and blue Mondays and parties and restaurants and bad moods and work and cooking and mirrors and rain and the flu and picnics and 4th of July and movie popcorn and birthday cakes and snowstorms and the scale and late-evening and mid-afternoon and gas prices . . . in other words, life?

Life is complicated, and evermore shall be. But you can integrate your diet into your life, and you can work out your life to be more compatible with your diet.

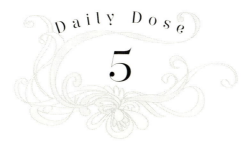

Daily Dose

5

What do my past dieting attempts tell me?

Well, if I just look at fifteen of them, one by one, they say I'm a total failure. They tell me I'm completely inept when it comes to the weight-loss challenge. They tell me I have no willpower or self-control. They tell me I will always weigh too much, I will always be too fat.

Except now I don't think like this anymore, because my 16th diet was a big, outrageous success.

What this tells me is, I didn't fail at dieting fifteen times; reaching my weight-loss goal was a journey of sixteen steps.

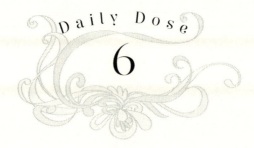

Daily Dose

6

What's the best greatest dieting trick ever?

Is it picking the ultimate best diet?

No.

Is it having a dieting buddy?

No. But that's a good one too.

Is it being perfect on a diet?

No.

Is it being not too restrictive?

No. But that helps.

Is it starting the diet on Monday morning?

No.

Is it taking pills?

No.

Is it exercising?

No, but that is a good idea.

Here it is: the best greatest dieting trick ever is learning how to STAY ON A DIET.

Staying on it is the tricky part.

Start by figuring out at least 5 things that interfered with your attempt to stay on a diet the last time you tried. Then come up with 5 brand new ways to handle those interfering things so they won't keep you from staying on the diet next time.

That's the idea, that's the trick. It's not really a trick at all. It's the smartest way to find weight-loss success.

And if you come up with 10 things that kept you from staying on last time, good. Figure out what to do about the 10 things. Or 20. Or even just 1.

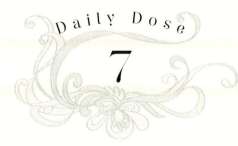

Y ou don't need to stick faithfully to your diet right off the bat.

Make as many mistakes as you can, all different kinds of mistakes. Consider this your training period.

Error management research shows that people perform better later when they have a training period where they are allowed to make mistakes. Trainees not only learn from their mistakes, they become better able to deal with the consequences of mistakes—things like frustration, loss of focus, and wanting to giving up.

Mistakes are always an important means of learning. So think of your mistakes in the early phase, the training phase, as positive and useful. Put aside what you learned in school, that mistakes are no good. With mistake training under your belt, you'll have less room for food and much more success dieting.

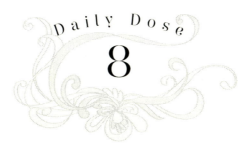

Daily Dose

8

Do you know your dieting ABC's?

Always go right back on when you fall off

Be mindful of your eating triggers

Consider every cheat a learning tool

Design a specific plan for getting through the rough spots

Enlist the support of those close to you

Focus on feelings along with food

Guide your diet process along a path of small goals

Hang on, even when you are not perfect

Imagine reaching your goal and how you will feel

Justify a cheat by carefully examining the situation where it happened

Keep your goals fresh by re-thinking them often

Lose weight, don't lose your mind

Make up your mind, and your body will follow

Navigate your way through holidays by easing up a little on diet rules

Organize the steps of your diet plan, but stay flexible

Prepare for the weight-loss journey before you take the first step

Question your negative, limiting beliefs about yourself

Remember other areas in your life where you successfully reached a goal

Stop and think before you automatically reach for food

Try again after you have a slip

Understand that defenses are at work when you try to change your behavior

Voice your feelings instead of stuffing them down with food

Work hard at resolving the non-food issues

X-out people and places that are conducive to overeating

Yes your way to your weight-loss goal with lots of mini-successes

Zero in on all your personal strengths

What good is the best diet on earth if you can't stick to it?

A 2005 study reported in the Journal of the American Medical Association showed that of the participants in four different diet plans (Atkins, Ornish, Weight Watchers, Zone) only 25% in each plan could stick to that diet.

If four major diets in a research study couldn't get 75% of people to adhere to their diet plans, how can you?

You need to figure out how to stay on a diet. The part of a weight-loss plan that helps you do this is the non-food part. It requires that you find ways to deal with whatever causes you to go off your diet.

You can make your own study of this. For example:

When you cheat, where are you most likely to be?

When you cheat, who are you usually with?

When you go off your diet, what kind of mood are you usually in?

When you go on a diet, when do you tend to give up the most?

What do you think are the personal issues that have made you a failure as a dieter?

Do you think you are involved in emotional eating?

Have you developed a way to deal with your feelings other than by eating?

What do you think would help you most of all to stay on your diet plan?

You see how the process would go. This is the kind of thoughtful analysis that will help you stay on whatever diet plan you choose.

There's the food part—and the *you* part. The *you* part is what really counts.

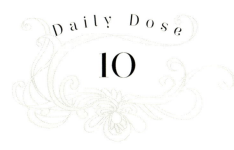

Daily Dose

10

Fell off that diet yet again?

Here's a wonderful exercise to help you.

Imagine that a best friend, or daughter, or sister, comes to you for advice about how to lose the 30 lbs she's put on over the last few years. She tells you she's tried everything she's ever heard of, and nothing works for her. She can't stick to it.

Imagine this person, and how deeply you care about her.

So, what would you tell her? What would you suggest? What would be your very best advice about how to do something so she could solve this weight problem she has that is making her so unhappy?

When you come up with your best, caring advice, write it down.

Then be your own weight-loss guru, and follow all of the advice yourself.

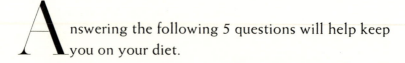

11

Answering the following 5 questions will help keep you on your diet.

1. *Did you pick a diet reasonable enough to follow?*
   If a diet is too strict, it can backfire. The gentler it is, the more likely you are to stay on it. There is great power in gentleness. If you are on a diet plan that is too harsh and restrictive, change to another one.

2. *Do you stay in tune with what you want for yourself?*
   Many times we set out to achieve a goal, but lose site of what the goal will do for us in our lives. Each week, refresh your memory about why you want to lose weight.

3. *Can you anticipate trigger situations?*
   These situations will definitely come up, and your best defense is to be prepared. Know beforehand what you'll be up against and make a good plan so the challenging situation won't result in a diet lapse.

4. *Can you think about weight loss as a journey of smaller steps?*
   When you set smaller tasks for yourself along the way
   to your final weight-loss goal, you gather successes.
   These successes give you a feeling of being capable,
   and that goes a long way toward helping you stick to
   your diet plan.

5. *What will you do after a diet cheat?*
   Cheating on a diet is something that throws many
   dieters completely off track. They think they need
   to be perfect, or it's all for naught. Not true. The
   best thing you can do to stay on your diet all the
   way to your weight-loss goal is to accept your cheat,
   and get right back on your diet. In this way, you can
   incorporate cheating right into your diet plan.

Y ou're desperate to lose weight; you go on a diet. Will you stick to it?

So many times a woman will begin a weight-loss plan with high hopes and determination, only to lose both along the way. And so many times it's a complete mystery why this happens.

Often, the "I will do it" is clear, up front, simple. You want to lose the weight, you want to change your bad eating habits, you decide to do something about it, you start. More hidden and complicated are the factors that work on you—from without and within—and get in your way.

It is not unusual for a woman to have absolutely no idea why she couldn't stick to it. Does this sound familiar? If so, why not go into your next attempt at losing weight acknowledging beforehand that this might happen.

And then what you can do is, BE PREPARED. Being prepared involves having a good plan to meet obstacles in advance of their appearance. It means not having just a flimsy positive attitude—ok, THIS time I'll really, really do it. It means having a new perspective on things to do to MAKE it happen the way you want it to.

And you know what? If you make a good plan, and then begin to falter, you will be able to see much more clearly what is making you falter. Well, I planned to do such-and-such, but this is what went wrong. Maybe now I can try this other way. You see? You would have your eyes and your mind tuned in. You would not just be going on blind faith.

Think, plan, stay tuned in, aware. That's how to do it.

Any woman who has been on a diet (every woman, no?) can tell you there is a big difference when it comes to being at the beginning of a diet, being in the middle of a diet, and getting toward the end of a diet. The dynamics change radically.

At the beginning of a diet, you are often propelled by high hopes, and the feeling of making a fresh start. You have energy, no mistakes to deal with yet, the excitement of doing something new and different, running on the jolt you get from taking off, like the starting gun of a race.

In the middle of the diet, it's not like that at all. It can be boring, it can feel monotonous, it can seem like there's no end in sight. This is a danger zone, and you need to find ways to keep on going. Your original motivating factors may be left in the dust, and you may forget why you're even doing it. This mid-diet time is critical, though, because it is the bridge that brings you from the starting gate to the finish line.

There are ways to re-motivate yourself, reignite the weight-loss fires within you. Don't let the middle-of-a-diet phase lull you into carelessly losing faith and giving up. You can find ways to traverse this longest part of the journey, if you put your mind to it. You can refresh your goals. You can reward yourself in new and different ways. You can take particular note of how far you've come. You can pay attention to the unique challenges you face during this possibly long, drawn-out time, and create effective ways to meet them.

When you are close to the end, it's different. Your goal reward is well within reach. There it is, waiting for you to claim it. That in itself will often rekindle motivation, and give you the final push you need.

Pay attention to every phase when you are trying to lose weight. Stay close to what you need, how you feel, what you do for and against yourself. Pay particular attention to these things when you are mid-diet. It may not have the pizzazz or glitter of starting and finishing, but it is the most crucial period of dieting time.

Losing weight is not always a feel-good story. As you probably know if you have ever lost weight, it can be uncomfortable, even painful at times. And it's usually not the eating part that's hardest. It's the emotional part.

Emotions get stirred up when you go about the task of changing your eating. That's what contributes to making things hard. So, how can you make it easier?

First of all, know about this before you even start. Anticipate it. Think about it. Be as ready as you can be for it. Don't expect that it will all go as you planned, like clockwork. It won't. You will be very pleasantly surprised to see how just being aware of the fact that it will get hard at times actually makes it easier.

If you have the mindset that you'll just pick an eating plan, go on it, and easily lose weight, you will run into unforeseen difficulties. But if you use your crystal ball to look into the future first, you'll be able to see that challenges lie ahead, especially "feelings" challenges. And then, of course, you can figure out ways to handle them.

Don't think you can get away from dealing with your feelings when you are trying to lose weight—there's no way. Instead, figure out how you can address them.

Use your head when you want to change your body.

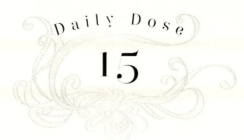
There is nothing as important when you're trying to lose weight as keeping an eye on your feelings.

Feelings.

You can eat them down, or you can jot them down and consider them.

It takes an awful lot of food to eat down your feelings.

It takes no extra food to write them down, and understand more about them.

Feelings are what make us human. Don't bury them.

Put these words up on your refrigerator. "Change is a process." This is something to believe in as you move toward your weight-loss goal.

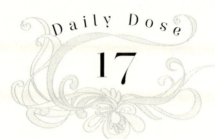

Daily Dose

17

I'm terribly sorry.

Oh, that's OK, you really don't need to apologize.

I just acted without thinking, totally. If I had stopped to think for a moment, it never would have happened. I didn't mean to hurt you.

I know that.

I don't know what comes over me at times like that. It's like I forget to think about you and your feelings and what's good for you. But I really do care about you.

We all make mistakes.

Yes, but what can I do to make it up to you?

Well, you said it. Just think a little more before you act. Think about what you're about to do, and if it's a good thing or a bad thing.

I will. And I just want to say, I like these moments of reckoning. Now we can go forward. I feel like I've wiped the slate clean. It feels great to be forgiven.

Even if you make another mistake, it's OK. I know you're trying. I have a lot of faith in you.

Thanks, that means a lot.

This was the gist of a conversation I had with my husband recently. I wrote it down afterward because I loved it and thought, why don't I talk to myself like that . . . especially when I cheat on my diet? Boy, would that kind of caring tone help me out.

Your aim is to lose weight. There are many ways of going about it, but any successful attempt at losing the weight involves some degree of thought. You can, of course, think about what you will eat in order to lose weight. But you can go much further in your thinking: you can self reflect.

How does self-reflection help you lose weight? Here's one way thinking about yourself—your actions and behavior and attitudes—can facilitate the weight-loss process. Suppose you were to look back at the end of each day on your diet, and reflect upon a moment in that day when you failed to act in a way that supported you in your weight-loss effort. This could involve eating off your diet, but it can also have to do with other thoughts and actions.

This is a way to monitor your behavior. By reflecting on your actions, or even your thoughts—especially if they're negative—you can see how you're really doing. If you do find that every day you do something—or many things—

that interfere with successful weight loss, couldn't you go about the task of changing those things?

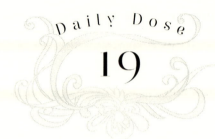

Daily Dose

19

H ow many calories in this fruits-of-the-forest pie, I wonder.

How many crazy self-critical thoughts are swirling around in my head?

If I eat chicken and salad for two weeks, that should be good for 10 lbs.

How come other women can do hard things, and I can't?

Something's wrong with this diet, it's just stupid.

I'm terrified by the thought of giving up my food.

I'll see if they have any diet food on the menu.

I'm ravenous.

Hey, I just found a "lose-15-lbs-in-3-weeks" diet on the net.

My heart is broken because I've disappointed myself one too many times.

Well, no use thinking about it any more, it's giving me a headache.

The real thoughts are often right there, waiting for you.

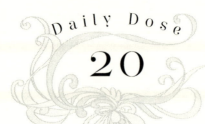

Daily Dose

20

The subject of high-risk eating situations has everything to do with sticking to a diet. Do you know what constitutes a high-risk eating situation for you? Do you know which situations pose the greatest risk to your sense of self-control?

The funny part about this serious subject is that high-risk situations in terms of eating can be different for different people. This is a story about two friends who decided to start dieting together. Here's how it went.

One friend did really well when she was at home. She ate pretty much everything that was on her food plan, felt satisfied, and didn't find it hard to stick with it. BUT every time she was out to eat somewhere—at someone's house or at a restaurant—she completely lost control. She ate much more than she meant to at these times, and ate things that were totally off the diet. And, actually, she thought she was doing well even then. She couldn't tell she was eating too much, but the scale knew better. And this happened pretty much every time she had a meal outside the house.

The other friend had a very different high-risk situation. She was most vulnerable to lapses when she was at home, especially when she was alone. Just being around food at home—just having certain things in the kitchen—could set her off into an overeating episode.

So, one of the friends needed to recognize how high-risk it was when she ate out. And the other had to acknowledge the trouble she had when she was at home.

So there you have it. Two women, both trying to lose weight, both facing high-risk eating situations, but the situations were exact opposites. They began to get a grip on this, first by admitting it to themselves, and then to each other, and then by helping one another prepare for the risky eating situation. The preparation was different for each one, as you may imagine. So while they were essentially dieting together, each had her own personal work to do.

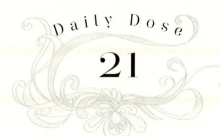

In the town is a street.

On the street is a house.

In the house is a kitchen.

In the kitchen is a refrigerator.

In the refrigerator is a freezer.

In the freezer is Chunky Monkey ice cream.

In my heart there's a hole.

And even though I know ice cream won't fill the hole, I go for it anyway, not knowing any other way to fill myself up. So I blow my diet.

And then I feel even worse.

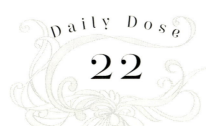

A very clever solution to feeling tempted is just this: *let the moment pass.* That's it, plain and simple. A moment is only a moment, and if you can let the moment go by without actually following your impulse to indulge, you may be very pleasantly surprised to find that the moment is only a moment; it doesn't last that long.

So, what is a moment of feeling tempted made of? There is a strong desire to have forbidden food. It may be right there in front of you, or it may be just the thought of something. You can call this a craving or an urge. You see the food, or you think of it, and you want it. You really want it, and you may have the feeling that you can't live without it right then.

If you get swept up in that kind of moment, you may not realize that you don't *have* to do that. You can actually do something different. You can let that moment pass, without acting on it.

To prove that you can do something different, try to let

a tempting moment go—just one time. See how it feels to not give in. Just do it once. Once is enough to show you that you can, in fact, do it. Then what happens is, the next time will be easier. You'll think twice about just going ahead and having the fattening food. You won't feel so compelled to do it because you'll have the memory of holding on until the moment passes. You'll be more open to what's possible in the situation. And it's safe to say that the third time will be even easier. Each time you are able to let that moment of temptation pass, it will require less effort. Over time, you might even become an expert at resisting temptation.

Everything worth doing takes practice to get it right.

Y ou can do it the easy way, or you can do it the hard way.

The hard way:

> Just pick a diet that sounds good to you and go from there. Leave all your bad habits and usual behaviors intact. Every time you run up against a destructive habit or an unwanted behavior that is ingrained in you, you will need to fight against it in order to keep to your diet plan. It's hard; it's exhausting.

The easy way:

> Take seriously the fact that no matter how good that diet is, some things you characteristically do will get in your way. These are the things to take notice of and work on. These are the things that need to change. If you address these habits and behaviors with careful attention, you can change

them. Then you can stop fighting against yourself, and that's when dieting becomes ever so much easier.

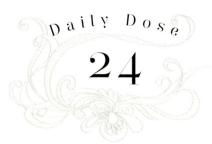

Here's what Ellie wrote when we asked her what she could and couldn't handle about going on a diet.

I can't handle

Starving

Obsessively counting calories

Eating different food than everyone else

Feeling cranky

Feeling deprived

Getting impatient

Feeling like I can't do it

The scale not going down

Other people's opinions

Getting discouraged

I can handle

Eating less than I'm eating now

Walking 2 times a week

Cooking something I love

Keeping a log of my feelings

Getting more rest

Asking for more support from my family

Taking it one day at a time

Then we encouraged Ellie to use each and every "what I can handle" idea and construct her plan around that.

She carefully took into consideration what she felt she could handle, and built herself a comprehensive weight-loss plan.

Her weight is still going down, the first real success she's had in a long, long time.

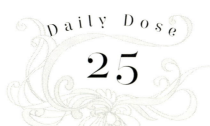

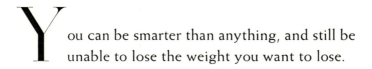

You can be smarter than anything, and still be unable to lose the weight you want to lose.

You can be a very accomplished woman, and still not be able to lose the weight.

You can be a very strong woman, and still not be able to.

You can be a woman of your word, and still have trouble when it comes to losing that unwanted weight.

You can be a great mother, and still not be able to get down to the size you're most comfortable in.

You can be a trustworthy friend, and still be unable to keep your promise to yourself to do it.

You can be a totally responsible individual, and still fall down on the losing-weight job.

You can be the controller of the family's budget, keeping everyone on track, and still be a diet failure.

You can be extremely talented in one or more areas, and still not be able to stick to it.

Sticking to it requires more than willpower.

It demands that you do the inside, personal-issue work you need to do.

If you are willing to consider this side of things, you will be all the good things you are, and also be that woman who can lose the weight.

Daily Dose

26

If someone gets married and divorced six times, you'd say she was doing something wrong, wouldn't you? Maybe picking bad partners?

If a woman starts a new business six times and each time it fails ultimately, you'd say she was doing something (or some things) wrong, wouldn't you?

If someone makes a recipe for beef bourguignon six times and each time it comes out inedible, you'd say she was doing something wrong, wouldn't you?

If a woman tries to fix a broken hot water heater six times, and it only works for a day or so before breaking down again, you'd say she was doing something wrong, wouldn't you?

So what do you say about a woman who has gone on six diets but still has not lost the weight she wants to lose?

Is that you?

Are you doing something wrong?

What?

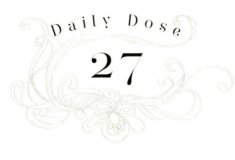

Measuring weight-loss progress doesn't only mean counting how many pounds you've lost.

Yes, the goal is to lose the weight. But if you focus only on the scale, you may miss some valid signs that you are really getting there.

The things to measure and concentrate on are your behavior, your old habits, if and how both are changing. Because once old eating habits begin to change, once that usual eating behavior of yours goes into transition, weight loss is bound to follow.

Keep a chart. Begin by identifying ways you act that you think most contribute to your being overweight.

Make a good plan for changing every one of those behaviors.

Take note of how well you are sticking to the plans.

This will tell you whether or not you are really on your way to goal.

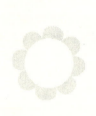

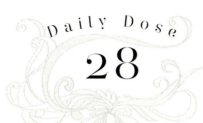

The ten commandments of dieting.

Thou shalt not abandon this diet without thinking it through

Thou shalt not give it anything less than a best effort

Thou shalt not eat unconsciously

Thou shalt not eat so little it hurts

Thou shalt not eat so much it hurts

Thou shalt not engage in self-deception about eating

Thou shalt not lose sight of the goal

Thou shalt not try and go it all alone

Thou shalt not take on too much

Thou shalt not give up

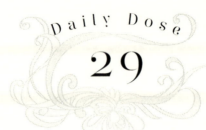
There you were, eating off your diet again. You didn't mean to, it just happened. Then you did it again. And before you knew it, you went back to overeating, and hating yourself for doing it.

Is there a way of inoculating yourself against such a chain of events?

There is.

Believe it or not, you can prevent such a chain of events from happening by practicing beforehand what you can do when you begin to slip. Actually, you can rehearse what to do so that when the time comes, you are prepared. It's just like rehearsing for any performance. You practice the rough spots over and over, and when the real performance comes, you have what it takes to sail right through them.

Working from a script might be just what you need to make your rehearsal time most effective. The script would define and describe the rough spots as well as the actions to take when the occasion arises.

Your plan of action should include what will be helpful to you at the time. Perhaps it will be dialog with another character (e.g., best friend, family member). It might also be "exit stage right" to get yourself out of the difficult situation.

Rehearsing for an upcoming difficult time when you might slip will give you the skills you need to get you through it.

And then you can give yourself the applause you deserve.

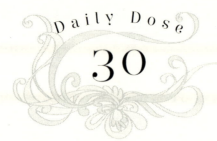

She comes through her front door, tosses her handbag down on the sofa, sits down and nestles in.

Tired. Drained. A bit lost. Low. Empty. Needing something. All in.

She needs something, but does not know what. She puts her feet up on the coffee table, hears voices coming from the family room, doesn't call out—not, hello! I'm home! Or—hi everybody! Just a silent, sinking-down moment, a complete and utter surrender to this late-day mood, which she feels head to toe.

She stays there, perfectly silent, not moving, not even re-settling herself, just staying exactly where she first plopped down. Jumbled thoughts come, a few tears, who knows why: a bad day, a hard month, very tired, defeated.

All this takes place instead of the old head-right-for-the-fridge that used to be her life.

After twenty minutes or so, she is ready, and calls out to everyone: Hi! I'm home!

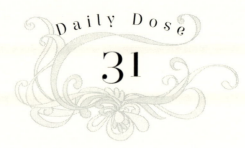

Daily Dose

31

ill me up

    fill me up, strawberry cheesecake

not because i'm hungry

because I'm empty

fill me up with your sweet richness

make me sweet

make me rich

make me forget all I do not have

enough love

enough self respect

enough achievements

enough courage

ease my pain, bite by bite

I'm counting on you

Here are some strategies to use when you lapse, slip, cheat, fall off—whatever you call it—while dieting. These are valuable strategies from *Relapse Prevention* by G. Alan Marlatt and Dennis M. Donovan.

Stop, Look, and Listen

First you need to stop whatever you are doing to look, listen and try to understand what is happening. Use the cheat as a warning signal. It says you are in danger. So just take a time out and see what emergency measures you can take.

Stay Calm.

You'll probably immediately feel guilty and self-blaming for a dieting transgression. That's OK—but then you need to let it go. Consider it a mistake from which you can recover.

Renew Your Commitment

A lapse has the potential to crush your weight-loss motivation. You think things like "it's no use". You might get hopeless.

So, set up an inner conversation between the side of you that wants to give up and chuck the diet, and the side of you that wants to keep going. And then remember: a single slip does not cancel out all your progress to date.

Think About What Led Up To The Slip

Quit blaming yourself as soon as you possibly can. Look at this slip as a specific, circumscribed event. Find out what things led up to it. Was it some kind of uncomfortable situation? Where were you? Who was there with you? How were you feeling? Why were you feeling this way? Then imagine the whole scene turning out differently. This time, imagine yourself coping with the situation much more effectively.

Here's the idea: a slip tells you something is going wrong that you need to pay attention to and fix.

Make An Immediate Plan For Recovery From the Lapse

Right away, get rid of anything that added to your lapse—for example, any tempting food. Or get away from the situation altogether if you can.

Leave physically if possible. Leave psychologically, at least for a few moments, to recover. Take some deep breaths. Relax. Try to settle your mind.

Ask For Help

If you are with people, ask for their advice to help you cope. If you are alone, you could call a friend or family member who might give you the support and assistance you need.

These are six powerful steps to take after falling off your diet. They give you the power to change what happens next. If you're used to dissolving into total eating chaos after a dieting slip, now you can repair the damage and continue dieting.

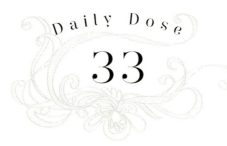

Daily Dose

33

Susan: And now to our feature human-interest story. We go into the middle of New York City where a real life drama is unfolding. A dieter is poised to jump off the diet cliff into the abyss. Let's go to our field correspondent, Dinah, who has the inside track . . . . Dinah? What's the latest? Tell us what's happening in this crisis.

Dinah: Yes Susan, I'm here with Jeannie who's trapped in her house, a victim of her own cravings and urges. They tell us all it takes is willpower, but here's Jeannie in the midst of this all-too-common dieter's dilemma— *what happened to my willpower?* Jeannie has always succumbed in the past. This time she's trying to resist, and that's why there's a crisis.

Susan: So, what is she doing right now?

Dinah: Well, it's sad to see, Susan. She's pacing back and forth between her kitchen and her living room, dialoguing with herself.

Susan: That must be quite a scene.

Dinah: Yes, it certainly is. Jeannie tells me that she's fighting not to add another notch to her belt. She doesn't want another diet gone wrong.

Susan: So Dinah, what happens now?

Dinah: Jeannie has agreed to stay on camera during this emergency. Let's see if I can get her in mid-pace . . . . So Jeannie, let's sit down. Can you tell me what brought on this present crisis?

Jeannie: I don't know, but suddenly I'm being held hostage by my kids' candy on the pantry shelf. Am I being a drama queen? I just feel torn apart. It's like this is the tipping point, one way or another. I don't know how to put out the fire. I did call my friend Sarah, but I got voice mail.

Dinah: So you needed someone to talk to.

Jeannie: But just because she didn't pick up, is that enough to push me over the edge? What am I not getting here? I really thought this time would be different. This new diet seemed like a great idea last Monday. But that's nothing new. I've been on every new diet since 1995.

Dinah: There's actually been no crime committed here against the diet yet, has there?

Jeannie: No, not yet.

Dinah: What would happen if you did fall off the diet?

Jeannie: I couldn't take it. It would be too hard for me. I couldn't tolerate giving up again. I'd feel like a total failure. You see? That's why I'm stuck. Why can't someone invent a diet you can stick to?

Dinah: Out of all those diets you've been on, not one was stickable?

Jeannie: Not one.

Dinah: What was wrong with them?

Jeannie: Nothing I guess. I just lost my willpower.

Dinah: Ah. That sounds like a universal problem.

Jeannie: It probably is. Where do you get the strength to hold on to willpower? I don't even know what willpower is. Is it one something, or is it everything you need to do to stick with it?

Dinah: Sounds like all those diets taught you something.

Jeannie: You have a point. I've read that most people don't kick any habit on the first try, or even the second.

Dinah: So what will your next step be?

Jeannie: I wish I knew.

Dinah: What do you think someone else might say about your ability to handle this crisis without giving up? What qualities would they see in you that could help you power up your willpower?

Jeannie: I'm a pretty strong person. I can withstand a lot without cracking.

Dinah: That sounds like what's needed here.

Jeannie: And I'm also resourceful. I can find things out . . . . You know, I could come up with a lot of ideas right here. I think I can get creative about this willpower thing, not let it die. Probably talking to my friend Sarah wouldn't have helped anyway. I love her, but she doesn't have an eating problem, so she doesn't really understand. But I do have a friend who lost fifty pounds last year. I've been too jealous to ask her how she made it all the way through, but it would probably help me to talk to her. You know, I'm feeling a little calmer now, and more willpowered. Do you know what I mean? I just thought of something else. I think my next step is to write these things down. Not my food this time—my thoughts.

Dinah: Sounds like the crisis is passing.

Jeannie: I think so.

Dinah: (to the camera) Well, we've averted a diet tragedy here. Not to say Jeannie will have a perfectly smooth ride from now on, but things are looking up.

This is Dinah, on location, Channel Twelve, Eyes on the Prize weight-loss news . . . . Susan, back to you in the studio.

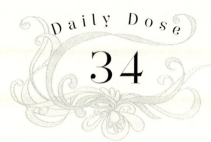

Daily Dose

34

Do you have unanswered questions about yourself and weight loss? Here are some possibilities of issues that may still be open.

How do I feel about my weight?

What goes wrong whenever I try to lose weight?

How do I feel about myself when I fail on a diet?

What does overeating do for me?

What does being overweight do for me?

Am I afraid to lose weight?

What am I afraid of most?

Do I go about trying to lose weight in the best way?

Do I give up too soon?

Do I blame others for my inability to lose?

Do I deal with my feelings effectively when I'm on a diet?

Do I expect to be successful on my next diet without knowing why?

Do I know what the best diet plan is for me personally?

Does my self-esteem suffer because I haven't lost weight?

Who can I count on to help me if I try again?

What do I need to do differently next time?

How would my life change for the better if I lose the weight?

What will I miss if I lose weight?

Are there questions here that sound important to you? If so, see what answers you come up with. Pay attention to these answers as you travel the diet road.

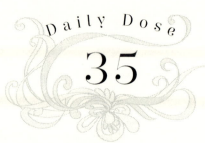

Daily Dose

35

Let's say you label yourself thus:

"I am a woman who can't stay on a diet." That's one way to look at it.

Now suppose you label yourself in a different way:

"I am a woman who very much wants to learn how to stay on a diet."

This is a whole different vantage point, isn't it? It leads you in a different direction. Instead of someone who *can't* do something, you are now describing someone who has a strong desire to *be able* to do something. All you've done here is change your focus. The slant is new. It's still the same you, but your new label allows for all sorts of possibilities.

You want to lose weight. You very much want to know how. You can probably already think of many things to do following this new concept of yourself. It is not just changing from negative to positive—it is more than that.

Because maybe by labeling yourself someone who can't stay on a diet, you've been putting yourself at a dead end.

The way you look at a problem has everything to do with being able to solve it.

Let's say you had a strong commitment at the start, and you've been into dieting, but as time goes by your resolve is weakening. What to do? Here are some methods people use to renew commitment in the middle of a diet.

Refresh your weight-loss goals. Restate them for yourself. Clarify them.

Review the areas of your life where weight causes problems for you.

Think about the consequences to your life if you don't finish what you started out to do. How will it be for you if you don't lose the weight?

Take a short vacation from dieting in order to come back to it with fresh energy.

Change the actual diet. Move on to something new and maybe better for you at this time (check with your physician to make sure it's a healthy way to go).

Join a weight-loss support group.

Ask for more help and support from people close to you.

Make a list of the personal strengths you possess that you can put harder to work for you in order to stay committed.

See which of these "sticking to it" methods work for you.

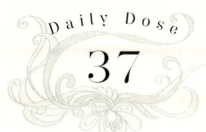
Plateaus are usually dreaded by dieters.

Reaching a plateau on the way to your weight-loss goal is to be expected. The task is to hold on to your motivation during a plateau.

Legend has it that King Solomon had a ring made with a saying on it that would always be true: "This too shall pass." Make yourself a reminder of this, like the King's engraved ring. Because if you can wrap your mind around the idea that the plateau is temporary—and also normal—then you can hold on. It's the feeling that it will last forever that makes you want to give up.

Remember: This plateau, too, shall pass.

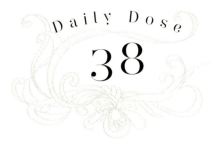
Do you know how to cheat and still make your diet stick all the way to goal?

Cheating on a diet is one of the most crucial aspects when it comes to success or failure. If you can handle those inevitable lapses, you will be overcoming an important obstacle. It is in this area of mistakes—cheats—where dieters' attempts can live or die.

Do you have what it takes to turn a cheat into a tool for success? Take this quiz and find out.

Can you pick up and go on with your diet after a cheat?

Do you stop to consider the circumstances surrounding a cheat?

Can you accept yourself as not being perfect on a diet?

Do you forgive yourself for a lapse?

Can you keep one cheat from leading you to another?

Do you believe that personal change is a process?

Do you think you will still be able to change the way you eat, even though you cheat sometimes?

Do you think mistakes are part of learning something new?

Can you avoid feeling like a failure because of a slip?

Do you think that changing your behavior might take more than one attempt?

Can you hold on to your self-confidence even after a cheat?

Can you forgive yourself for having less willpower at times?

Do you know how to include dealing with cheats in your weight-loss plan of action?

Can you avoid looking to a different diet just because of a cheat?

Can you avoid feeling guilty about a lapse?

Can you view a cheat as a small thing and not a catastrophe?

Do you know how to learn about yourself from your cheats?

Do you pay attention to what you do after you cheat?

Can you keep one cheating episode from turning into a total pig-out?

Do you still have hope after a cheat?

If you have more YES answer than NO answers, your chances of sticking with it are very good, even though you cheat sometimes.

If you have more NO answers than YES answers, you may be in danger of letting a cheat lead to a total collapse of your diet. Work on understanding your cheating episodes as much as possible—when they happen, why they happen, how often they happen. Use this knowledge and you won't have to give up.

One thing I know is that between a diet and real life there is a chasm.

I find myself too often standing in the middle of this nowhereville, grabbing at my life, pulling on the diet, trying to unite them. It's like oil and water. I try to shake them up together. I try to fold them in. I try to incorporate, but the two just won't blend. So I let go of the diet. Well, I can't let go of my life.

And yet, other women I know—busy, productive, ambitious women—can diet and lose weight. I've seen them do it.

What do they have that I don't have?

That's the question.

Daily Dose

40

Memories of past failures come into play when you start another diet. After all, no matter what diet you go on, you have to rely on yourself to stick to it. If you don't have a lot of experience with diet success, you probably don't have the feeling that you are capable of success.

Here's a way to feel more capable and have more belief in your stick-to-it ability. Think of something in your life apart from dieting that you've accomplished. It can be a big thing or a small thing, but it should be something important to you. Try to remember the process of achieving that goal. How did you do it? What were the steps leading up to it? How did you stick to your resolve to accomplish it? How did you feel when you got there?

Reminding yourself about how you were able to succeed in another area of your life is empowering. You can see how much strength you have to bring to a task. You can see that indeed you have creativity and problem-solving abilities. Then you can go ahead and bring these same strengths to bear on your problems with eating and weight.

When you are trying to kick a bad habit like overeating, sometimes it only takes a very minor blip to cause a major flip back into your unwanted behavior.

What a disappointment this can be for anyone who has been using good eating habits, dieting well, losing weight steadily, feeling good and confident.

Why a small blip can cause a major reaction is often hard to understand. But if you do have a relapse, investigate it. See what may have triggered it. Even the smallest things—a hurtful remark, a fleeting memory, a momentary loss of confidence, a passing negative thought—can be part of the mystery you need to solve.

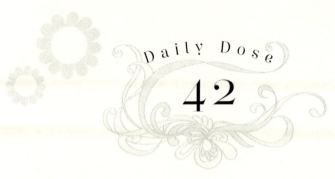

There are no dieting failures, only people who give up too soon.

What if you believed this with all your heart?

What would you do?

How would it make a difference for you?

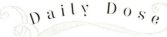

It takes less than a minute—sometimes even seconds—to blow a diet. Here's how to keep it together, stay on your diet so you can get to your weight loss goal. It only takes a minute, but it's that make-or-break kind of minute.

You don't need to keep falling off your eating plan. This one-minute act will give you the control you need to really stick to it.

It goes like this:

Slow down

Think

Open your mind

Pay attention

When you put together the first letters of each direction, it spells out **S-T-O-P**. This is how to STOP yourself from losing control when you diet.

1. ## Slow down
    A common reason people get into diet trouble is that they act on impulse. After all, you have probably trained yourself well to reach for food instantly without thinking about it. It's pretty much an automatic response at this point. A response to *what* is an individual matter. It might be a reaction to something distasteful or painful or hard or even just annoying. For some people it's even the way they respond to feeling good, proud or relieved. What reaching for food so automatically does is render you helpless, simply a creature of habit. You can very successfully interfere with this mechanism by first slowing down. You don't need to beat yourself up or take a hot bath or go for a walk. Just slow down, take a moment. That's all.

2. ## Think
    Here is where mind power comes in. During this moment when you have slowed yourself down, think about what's happening. Take a look around. Where are you? Who else is there? What's the situation? Is there something disturbing you about it? Is there something you need for yourself in this situation? Is there something you'd like to express? All these thoughts will serve to illuminate the problem of the moment. You are not just a victim of your habits when you exercise your ability to think.

3.   **O**pen your mind

     As thoughts come, be careful not to censor them.
     You might have thoughts that are surprising to you,
     things you didn't even know you think about. Maybe
     some are not such nice thoughts. Maybe you're really
     angry. Maybe you're feeling bad about yourself.
     Maybe a sad thought will pop up. In any case, try to
     let your thoughts come without closing your mind to
     them. They will hurt you much more if you ignore
     them.

4.   **P**ay attention

     Now that you've let your thoughts run a little more
     freely, pay attention to them. They will help you
     understand why you are teetering on the brink of
     blowing your diet. Pay attention to your thoughts
     at this moment even if they are small ideas, even
     if they don't seem significant to you. It doesn't
     necessarily take a great big thought to throw you
     off course. Quite often it's something small but very
     meaningful to you. The tiniest thought can be a key
     to understanding.

You will be amazed to see how well this one-minute diet
manager works. You will be interfering with your usual
reflex to eat, your usual habit of using food to control a
situation. Interfering this way will make its mark on your
unwanted habit and pretty much stop it in its tracks. Use

this one-minute diet manager again and again and you will change things for good.

So remind yourself next time you have the impulse to blow your diet . . . S-T-O-P.

Slow down

Think

Open your mind

Pay attention

Try it out. It only takes a minute.

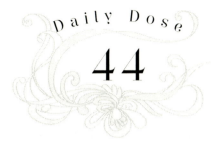
The first cookie tastes great—what a treat.

The second cookie is a triumph—I can eat exactly what I want.

The third cookie tastes like a little too much sugar.

I have to force down the fourth cookie.

The fifth cookie gives me heartburn.

The sixth cookie has no taste.

The seventh cookie makes me feel sick.

By the eighth cookie, I'm wondering what else I can grab to eat.

I have the ninth cookie while I'm thinking about having another treat.

The tenth cookie goes down and I wonder why, why did I eat all those cookies?

Why indeed.

45

When it comes to losing weight, "keep trying" is everything.

It's like a game of soccer.

The player tries, takes a shot on goal; it doesn't go in; she fails.

So she tries again, the keeper blocks it; once again it doesn't go in.

Then our tenacious striker tries again, and then again—no go.

But, you know what? The more shots on goal, the more likely it is she'll score.

The tries add up, and she scores at last.

Dieting is no different.

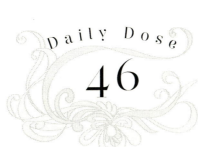

What many people do after they eat off their diet is to regret having done so. They feel guilty. They feel let down. They're angry with themselves. They feel trapped, because they can't go back and do it over again and do it right.

Since you can't change what's already happened, how about if you do the next best thing, which is to alter the effect of what's happened on the present. Let's see how you might turn a "looking back with regret" moment into a proactive moment.

Here's how it works. In the past, after falling off your diet and feeling terrible, maybe even hopeless about it, you probably said to yourself: If only I had done such and such, things would be better. The "such and such" might be: If only I had remembered my goal, or If only I had spoken up to that person instead of stuffing down my feelings, or If only I told my hostess I was dieting, or If only I skipped that luncheon with my friends, or If only I had given myself some "time-out" time and not gotten so tired. Anyway, you get the picture.

You are trying to retro-fix your regret, in a way, by thinking of something you could have done that would have been much better for you.

This is a great thing to do. Now you can tailor this "If only I had" thinking ever so slightly and come up with an alternative *future* action. This is the way to achieve a positive outcome next time, a better reality for you and dieting.

As a proactive strategy, you can take any "If only I had . . ." and transform it into a definite and positive plan. For example, instead of saying if only I had a piece of paper with me, you can say: I will bring a piece of paper with me next time I go out to dinner with a list of goals, and remind myself why I want to achieve them; I will prepare myself with satisfying things to say when I feel like someone is criticizing me; I will forewarn my hostess about the fact that I am dieting so she won't need to feel hurt if I don't eat much; I will skip lunch with my friends until I reach my goal and feel more confident; I will make sure not to get so tired that I can't focus.

You see how you can tool up with a plan like this? And it comes directly out of a regret. In fact, without the regret you might not know what you need to anticipate and plan for.

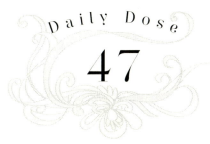
Y ou need it.

It's what makes it possible for you to override your impulses and resist tempting things you know you should resist.

You need it especially when you're dieting.

You probably lose it when you need it most. It just vanishes and leaves you hanging.

So what is it?

Self-control.

You most likely have it sometimes.

However . . .

Self-control is one of those things you can run out of.

When you're on a diet, the last thing you want is to run out of self-control.

So what can you do to make sure you have enough self-control to keep to your diet?

You can make sure you don't run out of self-control by squandering it, using it up elsewhere.

What does that mean?

You can make sure you don't use up all your self-control on everything else in your life when you're dieting.

For example, don't

> make a severely tight daily schedule for yourself
>
> be overly rigid about an exercise program
>
> spend too much time in social situations where you need to put on a false front
>
> be too strict with yourself about getting every little chore done

Self-control is necessary for losing weight. Make sure you conserve it so you have it when and where you need it.

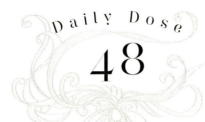

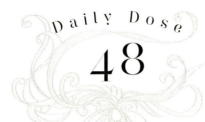

Daily Dose

48

N eed help sticking to a diet?

Change the rules.

Here are some rules you might be following, and ways to change them.

Old rule—Be perfect on your diet.

New rule—Factor in some cheats at preplanned times.

Old rule—Set your far-away weight-loss goal.

New rule—Start by setting a very small goal that you can achieve quickly. Then move on to another small goal.

Old rule—Wipe the slate clean by forgetting about all your past diet failures.

New rule—Remember past failure to see where you need to make changes.

Old rule—Be strong, and do it on your own.

New rule—Ask for help from people whenever you need it.

Old rule—Plan to reward yourself in a big way when you reach your weight-loss goal.

New rule—Reward yourself all along the way for small achievements.

Switch it out. Put in new rules for old, and see the boost it gives to your diet!

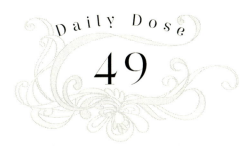

Daily Dose

49

Here's a question you might think is weird.

Are you emotionally attached to weight-loss failure? Before you simply dismiss the possibility, take some time to think about it. If you are, you can't possibly succeed at losing weight.

In the world of women and diets and weight loss, EMOTIONS RULE.

Y ou can un-stick your habits and stick-to dieting.

Sticking to a diet takes more than wanting to lose weight. It takes more than posting a food plan on the fridge. You need to have a plan for changing the things you do characteristically that bring your diet down every time.

Sticking to it is too hard when your behavior works against you. You can actually change what you do so it works *for* you. You may think changing your ways is too difficult, but you can do it. What it takes is recognizing that you do certain things without thinking, and these things continually get in your way. That's the trick. These are the things that cause you to fight against yourself when you are dieting. The good news: they keep their power over you only when you don't stop to notice them.

Here is a list of things you might do that have the potential to sabotage your diet again and again, no matter how good your intentions are. You probably don't have all of these habits, but even one or two can mean the difference between staying on and going off.

Which of these anti-diet habits do you stick to?

I hang out with people who overeat

I don't ask anyone for support when I am dieting

I try to be perfect

I put everyone else's needs first

I always expect to lose the weight fast

I don't speak up for myself

I never look in the full length mirror

I beat myself up for every cheat

I don't make time to relax

I engage in negative self-talk

I don't reward myself for my accomplishments

I don't prepare for high-risk eating situations

I don't admit that I have painful feelings

I blame myself for everything

I keep very tempting foods in the house

I don't get enough sleep

I take on too many tasks at one time

I set unrealistic goals for myself

I pick diets I don't particularly like

I never admit to myself how unhappy I am at this
weight

Take three habits you have that you think are the stickiest,
and begin to take them seriously.

For each one, ask yourself:

When does it occur most?

What purpose does it serve?

When did it start?

Are there other situations in my life besides dieting
where this habit comes into play?

Is this habit really necessary to my life?

Can I see myself living without it?

Would life be better without it?

You won't suddenly erase these habits from your repertoire
of behaviors, but believe it or not, the most important
thing is to notice them, admit them, acknowledge them.
This has a powerful effect. Take stock of the anti-dieting
things you do day after day without so much as a second

thought. Question these things, give them that second thought, think about them, and you will begin to un-stick them.

You deserve habits that work *for* you when you are dieting.

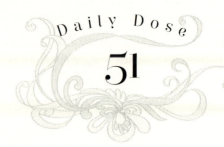

51

My biggest problem with eating comes around feeding the children.

They are six and four and they love lots of different kinds of food, including vegetables, fruit, as well as candy and chips.

I don't restrict them because I feel that wouldn't be fair. I just make sure there is enough good (nutritionally speaking) food around, and they really do go for it. Sometimes they choose fruit or yogurt over cookies for a snack. It's amazing, really.

I, on the other hand, crave the junk. When I have it around for them—like ice cream for dessert or something—I must have it. I can't help myself. That doesn't seem fair either.

It's like I become a child around food. Actually, my kids are more grown up about it than I am. They eat better, and they have no weight problems.

I think feeding the children brings up all my hungers—
know what I mean?

What is lurking right around the corner from a diet failure is the danger of losing your self-esteem.

Self-esteem: an evaluation you make about yourself, and an attitude you have toward yourself, which can be approving or disapproving. Self-esteem involves your own personal judgment—the extent to which you think of yourself as a capable person, a worthwhile person, a significant person.

Failure tends to make us feel inadequate and incapable.

Here's one way to prevent loss of self-esteem. Instead of pushing past diet failure out of your mind, call it up. Concentrate on exactly what happened. Don't automatically consider a past failure the result of some deep personal flaw or fixed shortcoming. Think hard about the circumstances:

Was it a good time in your life to diet?

Did you run into a relationship problem that you couldn't handle well?

Were you too strict with yourself?

Did you get enough support?

Were you able to give your diet effort daily emphasis?

Was the diet itself out of step with your lifestyle?

Did you give up too soon?

Answering questions like these immediately brings up new ways of doing things. For example, you can give your diet top priority now. Or you can enlist back-up support from friends or family. Or you can go a bit easier on yourself and allow for some mistakes, since no one is perfect.

It takes this kind of re-thinking to lift your self-esteem, which can put you right into success mode.

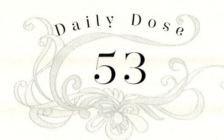

Daily Dose

53

I love food

I hate food

Food sets me free

Food imprisons me

When I eat a lot it lifts me

After I eat too much I feel low

I break my diet and feel powerful

I break my diet and I lose hope

Food gives me strength

I break my diet and feel like a weakling

Eating a lot calms me

Eating a lot upsets me

Food is my best friend

Food is my worst enemy

Admitting begets committing.

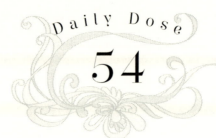

Do you START and STOP when you diet? Instead of stopping and starting the diet, here's your new stop/start list.

Stop—Blaming yourself for failing at losing weight

Start—Thinking about why you've been failing and what you can do differently

Stop—Trying to diet all by yourself

Start—Getting some help and support

Stop—Leaving it all up to the diet

Start—Putting your behavior up for change

Stop—Winging it

Start—Making concrete plans for what to do in difficult eating situations

Stop—Wanting speedy weight loss

Start—Concentrating on long-term change

So go ahead, START and STOP. But start and stop the
right things, so you can keep steady at your diet.

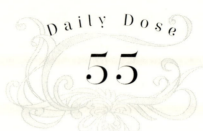

Daily Dose

55

Is there a chance you might be ambivalent about losing weight? Could that be one reason why you haven't been able to do it?

Why not explore your ambivalence. There are certain thoughts people sometimes have regarding particular issues that could be a result of ambivalence. If you pay attention, you might see that of course you want to lose weight, but you also don't want to lose weight.

Here are some thoughts that might signal how you are more conflicted about this than you may think.

I want to lose weight but . . .

I just don't know if I can do it.

I feel trapped in this weight gain, and I can't get out of it.

It's such a hard thing to do.

I feel deprived when I'm on a diet.

I have trouble fitting a diet into my life.

I'll probably just gain it back anyway.

I can't make food for everyone else and not eat it.

I have absolutely no willpower.

I'm confused about all the diet expert advice.

I never can diet in winter.

Thoughts like these may be masking ambivalence, conflict, the wanting to verses the not wanting to.

There's nothing wrong with being conflicted when it comes to losing weight. But if, underneath it all, you have a real desire to lose weight, it will help a great deal to think about the opposing side of you, and find out how you may be holding yourself back.

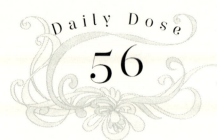

Y ou can walk a mile a day.

You can buy the latest diet book.

You can search the net for the latest weight-loss info.

You can listen to the experts.

You can start an exercise program.

You can make up your own diet plan.

You can do any and all of these things.

But: what is your "heart knowledge"?

What do you know in your secret heart, in your deepest of thoughts, in your most sensitive observations about yourself?

Heart knowledge—let yourself in on it.

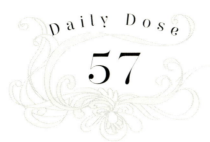

I went to my niece's wedding and I stayed on the diet all the way through, from 4 P.M. to midnight.

Here's what I realized by not focusing on food:

When I go to weddings, I feel like other people are happy and I'm not.

I always think I don't look as good as other women.

I'm very jealous of women who are thin.

When I'm not stuffing down food, I totally enjoy talking with people.

I feel better when I'm not full.

I like the feeling of being in control of myself.

I actually do have some willpower.

O ver in one corner of your brain: "Gotta lose weight. Gotta lose weight." Over in another corner of your brain: "I'm hungry. I'm hungry." Two warring factions. Even when a particular diet advocates food that is supposed to make you feel full, still an insistent message from that whispering corner: "I'm hungry. I'm hungry."

How do you make it so that "Gotta lose weight. Gotta lose weight." wins out over "I'm hungry. I'm hungry." One thing is, you could change the wording just a little bit, just a touch. Like, say, change the first to "I really want to lose weight. I really want to lose weight." And change the second to "I'm hungry, but I can withstand a little hunger. I'm hungry, but I can wait."

You can probably re-program lots of messages your brain has recorded over the years. They're just words, yes, but words can be oh so powerful.

Here's another corner of your brain talking: "I'm so fat, I'm a lost cause." Re-recorded, it might go like this: "I'm fatter than I want to be right now, but I have the power to change this."

Brainpower, thinking, mind/body connection, what it's all about.

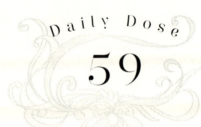

Daily Dose

59

Here is a way to objectify the experience of overeating, remove yourself somewhat, a way to step back and take a good look at what you're doing.

Right after an episode of eating too much, answer these questions:

What do you feel like physically?

What is your mood?

How were you feeling physically before you had this eating episode?

How was your mood before eating?

If your mood changed after eating, when exactly did it change?

How much did you eat?

What were you doing just before you went for the food?

What were you doing one hour before you went for the food?

Instead of simply trying to rule yourself into not overeating, give yourself the opportunity to step away from the behavior a little bit, and be more objective. Give yourself some room to think about it.

Demanding of yourself that you suddenly quit a self-destructive behavior usually doesn't work. But if you give yourself time and space to examine it, you've achieved a very important step toward stopping the behavior. The time and space allow for greater understanding, and for the possibility of doing something different in the future.

The very best way to keep a behavior is to let it continually run on automatic, and never stop to think about it.

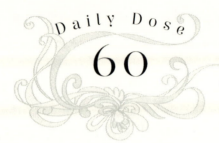

Daily Dose

60

Last year, I did more than just decide to lose weight. I realized that I wasn't living according to my own values. I asked myself, *what kind of women do I admire most?*

The answer:

women who are honest

women who are creative

women who are giving

women who are smart

women who are compassionate

women who are in touch with themselves

It was clear that my eating and my weight were interfering with my own expectations and desires for myself. I wasn't living up to some of my own benchmarks for being the kind of woman I admire. With that in mind, I went on a diet. My attitude was good. I was high on this new reason for losing weight.

Not that it was easy breezy—there were very tough times. But the power struggle was gone. I wasn't fighting against it. When things got hard, I found a way around them, because I wanted to. I knew I was doing something important for myself. I was becoming the woman I wanted to be, an honest woman, a compassionate woman, a woman who is in touch with herself, someone I could feel really good about.

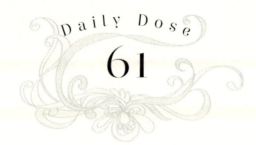
I've been sticking to a pretty rigid financial budget, as so many are. None of us knows what lies ahead, right? Even big Wall Street players are suffering. So a good budget, where you keep account of how all your money will be spent, seems appropriate. I figured it would keep my family from overspending, and it's working.

So after about the first month, it dawned on me that I could do the same thing with a diet—stick to a budget.

I know this is not a new idea, but the way I framed the idea was new to me. I've always followed the experts about how to eat to lose weight. Some say one thing, some say the opposite. We all know how it goes. The advice changes every day.

This time, I decided to simplify and get down to basics. I figured out that for my height and body type, about 1500 calories a day would be a good plan for weight loss. My doctor agreed.

So I simply went with the 1500. At first I thought, well if I don't cut out all sweets, and bread, and potatoes, I'll just eat them all the time, and I won't be healthy. But that didn't happen. I naturally gravitated toward a good mix of foods, and even some candy bars here and there (my weakness). My only requirement was to know how many calories I was eating, and each day they needed to add up to just about 1500.

The thing is, this has freed me. The main thing making a difference is that I am following my own advice, and it has empowered me. I always felt like a little girl when I was on a diet, doing what someone else was telling me to do. Now I feel like I am in control, because I am making the decisions. And then, most important of all, I am free to pay more attention to things that get me wanting to eat too much. I have more time and energy to consider my feelings, while before I was full force trying to follow the diet of the week, paying attention to every little detail obsessively.

Calculating calories is a cinch for me. It only takes minutes. Figuring out what really makes me eat too much requires more. Now I have more to give to that.

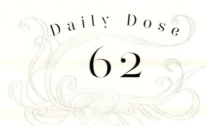
B elieving that you can lose weight counts—a lot.

Did you know that if you believe you will succeed at something, you are more likely to:

exert greater effort

regard errors as learning experiences

persevere for longer

be less distracted by anxiety, frustration, and self-doubt

If you are on a diet, and if you think you are a non-believer in yourself, see what you can do to change that.

Dieting sucks . . .

But it doesn't have to!

Here are 10 DIETING DON'TS that will make the whole experience much happier:

Don't

waste your energy on any diet that makes you starve

set your weight-loss goal at 5 lbs per week. Make it more like 1 to 2 lbs per week

expect weight loss to happen one-two-three

be afraid to try a different diet if the one you picked isn't working

try to hide the fact that you're dieting from people close to you

get too obsessive about weighing yourself

give up after a cheat—keep trying

set your ideal weight goal impossibly low

If you can follow these "don'ts", you can actually bring dieting out of the "it sucks" category and make it a much more enjoyable challenge. And the more enjoyable it is, the more likely you are to stay with it.

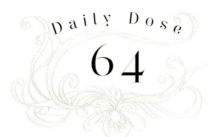

Daily Dose

64

Hang tough!

I am hanging tough. How much tougher can I possibly hang?

I'm sorry. I didn't mean to be pushy. It's just that I want the best for you. You're doing it, and I'm rooting for you.

There is one thing you can do for me.

What's that?

You can go easy on me when I run out of willpower.

Of course.

Please don't make me feel guilty, or foolish, or like a failure.

I won't do that.

It's just that when I lose my resolve, I can't tell who's a friend and who's a foe. I'm so extra-sensitive about everything. I hope I make it this time.

I hope you do too. I love you, you know.

Thanks, that really helps.

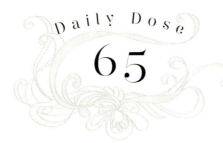

When I let go of the scale, I started to let go of the weight.

I know it sounds like a trick, but that's exactly what happened.

My whole adult life, I've used the scale as a kind of control center. I would obsessively get on, whether I would be on a diet or not. If I wasn't on a diet I'd get on three times a day to see how bad it was, how much I was gaining. If I was on a diet, I'd get on three or four times a day to check if the diet was working.

Needless to say, if I didn't lose weight every day, I'd lose heart and ditch the whole thing.

And if I gained anything, I'd tell myself it's no use anyway, so I might as well just eat.

So I took the scale and plunked it right into the garbage, and I swore I wouldn't buy a new one.

I am still on my diet. I know the weight I started at, but not exactly how much I've lost. But I am down at least one size in six weeks, and my really fat clothes are hanging off me. I can't believe it myself.

Try to remember, there is a difference between a simple slip and a total collapse. This is one of the most important pieces of information you can keep with you when you are dieting.

A slip is a single instance of going off your diet. It is not a complete return to your problematic eating behavior, and you don't have to let it get to that.

Don't do it. Take the slip and use it as an occasion for learning. That is how to avoid a catastrophic collapse of your whole weight-loss effort.

Yes, of course your goal is to stay on your diet as much as possible. But no one can be absolutely perfect, not for any length of time, anyway. So when you make a mistake, don't compound that mistake. Don't equate the one slip— or two or even three—with total failure.

When you do slip, see what happened, hold your head up, and get on with it. Each time you figure out a slip, it will lessen the chances for another slip. Each time you figure out a slip, it makes you stronger.

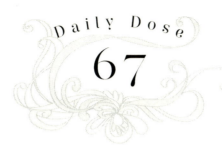

Everyday things that can wreck your diet (if you let them)

an unexpected change in schedule

a scare

a snowstorm

a very bad day

hurt feelings

a higher-that-expected scale read-out

a skinny friend

a shopping trip

a critical remark

a restaurant dinner

an argument

self-criticism

a disappointment

an old habit

a failure

fatigue

a small weight gain

impatience

the mirror

a temptation

feeling lonely

a negative thought

feeling deprived

There is not one thing on this list that you can't prepare yourself for, plan for, think out, feel out, and find your way through *without* giving up your diet.

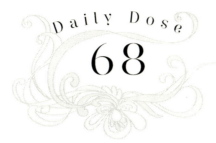

Daily Dose

68

It doesn't make sense. You went on the best diet ever, so why aren't you thin?

Well, beneath the surface of your common sense world lies another world.

The answers to weight-loss success rely on your common sense, but also on your deeper sense of things.

To unlock some of the secrets of why you haven't yet been able to resolve your food and weight issues, you need to use common-surface sense, along with that deeper sense. If you've had a rocky time of it—dieting, losing, gaining back—combining the two levels of understanding will allow you to solve the mystery.

Common sense may say:

"I shouldn't eat that."

While just beneath that thought is another:

I'm very angry right now—help.

Common sense may say:

"Everyone is doing this diet, so it must work."

While just beneath that thought is another:

I'm not as good as everyone else.

Common sense may say:

"I'll have some more, but just a little more."

While just beneath that thought is another:

I hate to deny myself.

The common sense thoughts come in handy, for sure. But the ones just below the surface have a lot more to do with dieting success or failure. They're the ones to get hold of, explore, and understand.

When Babe Ruth was asked why his salary was more than the President of the United States made, he replied, "So what kind of a year did he have?"

So . . . what kind of a year—weight-control wise—did you have?

Think back over the last twelve months, especially if you are in a place where you don't want to be with your weight.

What kinds of moves did you make over the last twelve months to help you lose the weight? And most importantly, did they actually work?

You can use the past year as a testing ground. Figure out where you went right and where you went wrong. Keep the right moves in your repertoire—the ones that were effective—and eliminate the wrong moves that got you nowhere.

That's what a journey toward any of life's accomplishments is—you adjust, readjust, change, alter, re-start, learn, gather information, evaluate, analyze, and above all: TRY AGAIN.

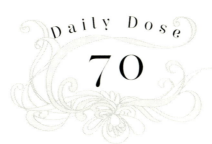

When Sunday comes, and there's nothing planned, that's when I battle eating the most.

Sunday can be fun, blue skies, but when it's quiet with no people around, I grab food.

I don't know, the day stretches out in front of me seeming endless, and I can't think what to do with it.

Then, of course, there's always the idea in the back of my mind that the next day is Monday, dieting day, so it doesn't matter what I do on Sunday.

It's just that on these empty Sundays, I like to fill myself up. I'd love to find another way to do it.

For many women, boredom is a big trigger for losing willpower. But what you call boredom may be simply a stretch of un-busy time when you don't know what to do with yourself. So eating comes to mind.

There are a thousand things you can do besides eat. Think about what you might do during these open-ended periods when you aren't obligated to do any specific thing.

What would be pleasurable for you? What do you love to do?

Boredom means different things to different people. You might feel a bit anxious by actually being free to do as you please. You might be keeping the thought in the back of your mind that you are shirking some responsibility or other. You may not have a good sense of what you'd really like to be doing.

Dealing well with "boredom"—calling it what it really is— can solve a great big dieting problem.

No one wants to lose something close to them.

So what are you in danger of losing when you start dieting, besides the weight?

There is something you will surely lose if you are successful with your dieting and start to lose weight— living life the way you have been used to.

Leaving behind your problematic eating and your state of being overweight will, besides bringing you joy, probably cause you discomfort. It's human nature. This is why self-change is not so easy.

Changing anything important about yourself can alter your sense of security because you are losing part of your self. But change is very definitely possible, despite the discomfort and loss you may feel. You can get through the discomfort in order to change for the better.

Remember to be aware of the discomfort you may experience along with changing. It might come in the form of anxious thoughts and feelings, or in conflicting thoughts and feelings, or in moodiness, etc.

If you feel that you can't face your discomfort alone, it's understandable. There are support groups, counselors, and therapists who are very knowledgeable about these matters. You can always get help if you need it.

Daily Dose

73

Scientific researchers who study how the universe works don't shoot directly for a grand goal. They focus on bite-sized problems that seem relevant and solvable. This methodology pays off, and scientists are able to make small steps toward solving the big fundamental questions.

Losing weight works the same way. The best thing to do is begin by solving some smaller issues related to weight problems. For example, instead of trying to solve the big picture, "why can't I lose the weight", start small by asking "why do I go off my diet when I _____ (example: visit my sister)?"

You can then address this circumscribed problem and come up with an answer and a solution that are very workable.

If you can proceed this way, tackling your "bite-sized" weight problems, solutions will add up. Each smaller weight problem solved will be a step toward solving the big question, "why can't I lose the weight". All the in-between steps make up a path that brings you to that big problem solved.

Message: *start small*.

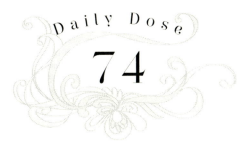

I max out my credit cards.

I max out diets too.

What do I mean?

I push it to the limit. If it says have 25 points, I have 25 points, and push just a little farther, figuring I'm still in the ballpark. If it says have a fist-size portion, I make the biggest fist I can make to measure. If it says 2 to 3 fruits a day, I have 3 and then maybe a part of a 4th, telling myself fruit is good for you. If it says veggies are a freebie, I'll have 10 cups of veggies. If it says only 1 cup of coffee, I have 1 giant mug. If it says artificial sweetener is allowed, I'll put in 5 packets. If it says allow yourself 1 free meal a week, I make sure that meal is packed with calories, start to finish.

Maxing out is something I need to quit.

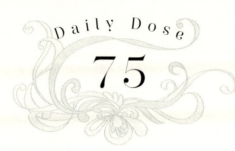

Daily Dose

75

If I were thin, I'd glide like a dancer.

If I were thin, I'd walk into the room and all eyes would be on me.

If I were thin, I'd prance before my mirror, trying on gorgeous outfit after gorgeous outfit.

If I were then, I'd look twenty years younger.

If I were thin, I'd wear a two-piece.

If I were thin, my friends would look up to me.

If I were thin, I'd be a better person.

If I were thin I'd be a success.

If I were thin, there'd be nothing else to want.

If I were thin, all my problems would be gone.

Can you count on getting thin to fix everything? Do you know in your heart of hearts it can't possibly—and does that get in the way of doing it?

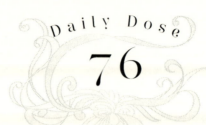

D-I-E-T

D is for how I DON'T want to be overweight any more

I is for the INSIGHT I'm gaining about why I haven't been able to stick to any diet

E is for ENERGIZING my life with self-knowledge

T is for TRYING again with this new outlook

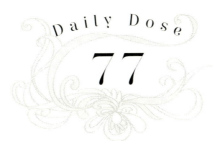

Y ou'd be surprised at how important positive self-
statements are.

Try this out.

> Say out loud to yourself: I just can't lose weight.
>
> How does this make you feel?
>
> What do you think of yourself when you say this?
>
> What thoughts follow after you say this to yourself?
>
> What do you think this statement would lead you to
> do next?

Now try this out.

> Say out loud to yourself: I haven't been able to lose
> weight yet, but I'm going to figure out how to do
> it.
>
> How does this make you feel?

What do you think of yourself when you say this?

What thoughts follow after you say this to yourself?

What do you think this statement would lead you to do next?

There's a world of difference between the two. Your mind is very receptive to what you say to yourself. Be careful.

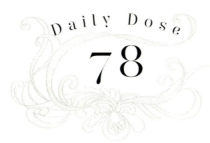

C*ueing* can help you get through a dieting roadblock.

Use a word, a gesture to yourself, a strong thought.

You need to develop cues beforehand. They are reminders to yourself. Using them can become a ritual. Cues can mean the difference between sticking to a diet and not sticking to it.

Here's one way they do it in sports, and it works every bit as well when you're trying to achieve a weight-loss goal.

Picture a time when you were on a diet and you were able to resist a temptation. Think of how it felt to resist the temptation. Remember just how it was to do that. Remember exactly how it made you feel to stay right with your personal goal.

Then you come up with your cue. It could be a quiet "you go girl" or "now you're really getting there" or "excellent!" or "yes!". It could be a vision of yourself in those jeans you're dying to get into again. It could be giving yourself a literal pat on the shoulder.

Whatever the cue is, it will represent that moment of dieting triumph. Pick one cue, and practice pairing the cue with the memory of a successful moment. Try to make your cue short and sweet, not too complicated, something you can call upon to do and say at a moment's notice.

So let's say you're up against a difficult moment. You can then give yourself your rehearsed cue, and use it to recall those feelings of success. It will be your signal to act that way again.

You need some handy, dandy dieting tools. This is a good one.

Buying the latest diet book is always easy. But soon the terrain becomes steep and treacherous. The first glimpse of trouble usually happens at around the second week mark, I don't know why.

What happens is, I start to translate my mood—good or bad—into an eating episode.

I'm at that point right now. I see myself doing this and it feels very familiar.

Like yesterday, when my daughter didn't come home. She's sixteen, so I really was worried. When she finally walked in the door, I was, needless to say, relieved and happy. I went straight to the fridge. But for some reason I stopped in my tracks. I asked myself, *what in the world does going through the fridge now have to do with my daughter's safe return home?* I couldn't think of one reasonable answer, so I closed the refrigerator door.

I was glad I did it, but it felt strange. It wasn't what I do. It wasn't me.

But it told me something. One of the things I don't like is feeling strange.

Are you in trouble when it comes to keeping up motivation?

There is a method that can help you. It's called the awareness-of-rationalizations technique developed by H. Reed and I. L. Janis. The research was done with smokers, but it easily adapts to people who have eating problems.

The basic idea is to eliminate some of your rationalizations that lead to weight-loss failure.

Here are eight rationalizations for overeating and staying overweight:

1. No one has proved that being overweight is really so bad for you.

2. The only big health problem is heart disease; my heart is fine.

3. I've been overweight for a long time, so it's probably too late to do anything.

4. If I eat too little, I'll be an anxious wreck.

5. Overeating is an unbreakable habit for me.

6. When I diet, I get too irritable.

7. It's my business if I'm overweight—I'm not hurting anyone else.

8. You only live once, might as well enjoy it.

NOW ASK YOURSELF THESE QUESTIONS:

Have you ever used any of these excuses?

Have you ever thought any of these things?

Do you see these arguments as valid?

Have you ever heard anyone else use these excuses?

Do some research. Find some personal and factual arguments that counter any of the rationalizations you may use.

In the Reed and Janis study of smokers, the technique of opening up and examining people's rationalizations about their problem behavior was a significant force in helping them quit.

Almost every woman who has tried to diet has failed at one time or another. Diet failure is often triggered by stress. This probably doesn't come as news, but it's worth thinking about again.

Here's another fact that isn't so obvious. Stress does not appear to make people eat more if they are NOT on a diet. It isn't that stress simply makes everybody hungrier as a general rule. Rather, what seems to happen is that stress loosens the self-control that a dieter in particular has been trying to hold onto. Stress tends to weaken inner restraints. Therefore, people who are on a diet tend to eat more when under stress.

Coping with stress, whether it is an everyday pressure, a relationship problem, a career setback, or something bigger and bolder like severe trauma, often results in a breakdown of willpower. And here's another fact you might want to keep in mind: Most major willpower breakdowns happen late in the day, after people have gone the longest without sleep. Dieters mainly go off their diets in the evening.

So, spare yourself as many tempting situations as possible, both after a stressful situation, and also in the evening. The effort you put forth in dealing with stress can be depleting. If you are depleted, and then faced with being tempted, the likelihood is you will not have enough strength to resist.

So you can try, to the best of your ability, to spare yourself from having to exert too much willpower in the aftermath of stress, and after a long day. Put yourself in a position at these times where you are not exposed to cues or opportunities that might require you to have a lot of willpower. Try to create a temptation-free zone at these crucial times.

Here's something to consider: The choices you make about what and how much you eat depend in large part upon the behavior of your eating companions.

Social influence on your eating is very powerful. It is so powerful, in fact, that it can override any weight-loss goals you have set for yourself.

Analysis of social influences on eating indicates that people actually use how the people around them are eating as their guide. This makes no sense when you think about it. Why abandon your diet just because someone else is eating a lot? But that is exactly what people tend to do: follow the example of others.

This works both ways. Someone who is in the presence of others who are eating modestly tends to "downsize" her eating.

So the question is, who do you hang out with when you are dieting?

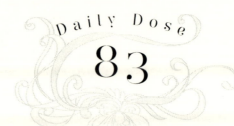
Do you know about being a good listener?

Here are things a good listener doesn't do:

She doesn't ridicule or label

She doesn't lecture

She doesn't judge

She doesn't blame

She doesn't threaten

She doesn't moralize

She doesn't command

She doesn't change the subject

She doesn't criticize

She doesn't issue orders

Be a good listener when you talk to yourself. Be open. Appreciate. Encourage. Take your time. Be respectful. Be flexible. Be attentive. Be accepting. Listen well to yourself, and it will help you lose weight.

I'm taking an experimental journey.

I like winners, but I'm not a winner when it comes to losing these same, hanging-on, 25 pounds. Oh, I've lost it, but I always gain it back.

Here's the experiment. Every time I cheat I will ask myself one question: What is making me go off my diet?

Instead of always plotting that tomorrow I'll do better, or I'll make up for the cheat by skipping a meal, or maybe I better wait until after the summer, or after Christmas, or after the weekend, whatever, I'm going to do it another way. I won't try and figure out how I can diet better. I'll make a study of how, when, and why I keep blowing it.

That's what I call an experiment.

In order to make a breakthrough toward any goal you are pursuing, you need to keep hanging around in the right neighborhood. What does this mean?

Well, it means immersing yourself in the problem, trying out solutions, thinking about it, being open to new ideas about it, trying out new routes to getting there, learning from mistakes, refining future efforts. All of this greatly increases the likelihood that you will have a breakthrough and reach your goal.

Basketball players know that in order to score, they need to keep hanging around in the areas where they make their best shots. A player may be off his/her shot in one particular game, but it's continually being there, in the right place, attempting those shots again and again, that eventually pays off in points scored.

It's the same with movie stars. Often we'll see a hit movie with a lead actress we've not heard of before. We might think of her as an overnight success, but this is almost never true. She has most likely:

Gone on countless auditions

Lost roles to other actors

Taken many acting classes

Watched lots of movies

Taken some very minor roles

So keep hanging out in weight-loss country.

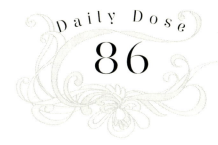

Janie: I don't know about you, but I just ate a whole cantaloupe.

Clara: That's nothing. I ate two sleeves of Oreos. Double stuff.

Janie: I woke up in the middle of the night and finished Amy's birthday cake.

Clara: I polished off the pot of mashed potatoes, then I drank the gravy.

Janie: I went through the Dunkin Donuts window twice, once for a bagel, then for donuts.

Clara: There was nothing in the house, so I melted a bag of chocolate chips and ate it with a spoon.

Janie: I finished the last drop of Honey Bunches of Oats and the kids had no breakfast.

Clara: I popped the button on my biggest pair of pants.

Janie: I'm wearing Justin's size 36 jeans.

Clara: Nothing in my closet fits.

Janie: I feel awful.

Clara: What happened to our diet?

Janie: What always happens.

Clara: I don't think these weird contests are helping us.

Janie: You mean who can be the worst. It's really dumb.

Clara: Let's cut it out.

Janie: I will if you will.

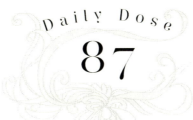

Daily Dose

87

D o you know one of the worst things for you and your diet? It's all-or-none thinking:

Totally on a diet or totally off a diet

Being totally good or being totally bad

Totally good foods or totally bad foods

Being totally perfect or being a total cheater

Totally starving or totally stuffing

Total success or total failure

The world isn't black and white, and neither are you.

Each of these opposites has gradations. For example, you can be on your diet but go off it from time to time. Still, you can consider yourself on a diet. Remember that change is often two steps forward one step back. You can think of a few weight gains as acceptable while dieting.

Also, weight-loss success doesn't come all at once at the end. You can count up the smaller successes and be triumphant even before you reach your ultimate goal.

All-or-none thinking is most definitely a dieter's enemy.

E ven when your diet backfires, it can still be saved.

A big risk for having your diet backfire is if it is too restrictive This can mean too restrictive in terms of the actual calories you take in; it can be too restrictive in the type of food it allows—like all protein or all carb; it can be too restrictive about when it allows you to eat or not eat; it can be too restrictive in the actual meals that make up the plan, dictating exactly what each meal should consist of; it can be too restrictive in dictating the method of cooking allowed—only boiling, only steaming, no frying or sautéing.

Any one or more of these restrictions can cause a backfire. It is human nature to rebel against being too constrained. So if you find yourself rebelling against your diet, it would be good to go over the plan itself. Consider whether it is too limiting for you. Even if it promises weight loss, it won't work if it's too hard to stick to.

There are a number of things you can do to remedy this

situation. You can of course, always look around for a less restrictive diet, or you can loosen the rules here and there so you can tolerate it better—it's your choice.

Don't be too drastic; it almost never works. And don't give up! Make the necessary adjustments, and forge ahead.

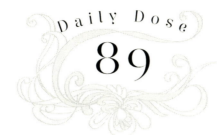

Weight loss is all about achieving your desired end goal. But what you have to do to reach your end goal can be terribly difficult, especially if you have to wait a long time for your reward.

Thus, it behooves you to have sub-goals for yourself. By having sub-goals, you partition the weight-loss journey into smaller tasks, which makes the journey much less difficult. With sub-goals there is the potential for each task you complete to bring its own reward. You don't have to wait all the way until the end.

Probably the best reward you can get from completing a weight-loss task is seeing that you are making progress. Seeing progress gives you the encouragement you need. Feeling encouraged is what will get you through all those difficult self-changes you are making.

Sub-goals, rewards, acknowledging progress, and feeling encouraged are the stepping-stones to your weight-loss goal. Don't make yourself wait all the way until the end. It's not fair.

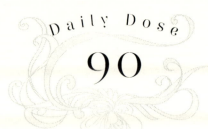

90

Set the mood for dieting.

Create the aura around you, make it conducive. Give yourself the right milieu.

For example:

Can you stick to your diet with all kinds of tempting sweets in the house? Well, intellectually you may think you should be able to. But if your instinct tells you no, then clear the shelves.

Are all your friends overweight, real big eaters, not successful losers? Is spending a lot of time with them conducive to dieting? If not, cut down.

Is your life very noisy—no quiet "you" time? Is this the atmosphere that perpetuates the diet mindset? Probably not.

How is your exercise quotient? It's not that exercise necessarily makes you lose weight. The value of exercise while you diet is how it makes you feel, not only physically, but mentally. It can lift your mood and contribute to the feeling that you can accomplish things, things that are good for you. This will spill over into dieting.

Are there "blue skies" in your life? do you have enough good times? This is a serious matter. Make sure your days and weeks are balanced out with as much enjoyment as hard work and responsibilities.

It's in your hands.

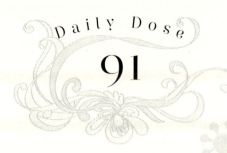
I stopped trying to look like my sixteen-year old daughter. No babydoll tops, no spaghetti straps. Last year I turned forty, and it was my turning point.

Maybe one day I'll do Botox, or even get a little eye job. If I want to at some point, then so be it. But for now, nothing like that.

I let go of avoiding the mirror. This is me.

I stopped trying to create the ideal persona and then struggling to live up to it.

I let go of the blame game. It's not my husband's fault, or my life as a juggling act.

I let go of trying to be something I'm not, which can't be done.

I stopped hating myself.

Then I lost a ton of weight.

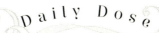

Daily Dose

92

Losing weight seriously involves the psychological side of things. But that doesn't mean the environment is left out of the equation—far from it.

Let's say you are on a diet, trying hard. First, picture yourself at home, with all your handy diet foods in the fridge, perhaps a pair of "skinny" jeans hanging on your closet door for inspiration, maybe a friend coming over for lunch who's also trying to lose weight, your food log and feelings diary close at hand. All this goes to make a supportive, encouraging environment, doesn't it?

And now, picture yourself at a restaurant that has yummy food on the menu. It's your friend's birthday celebration, and everyone is partaking of food and drink to take full advantage of the party and have the utmost good time. No one would expect you to stick to a diet here, right? There will be a big cake for dessert, there's lots of wine flowing, and you feel all loosened up. And to eat a skimpy portion of fish and salad and skip the cake altogether would make you feel like a party-pooper.

Which situation will help you lose weight?

It's the negotiating you do between your inner (emotional) and outer (environment) worlds that is crucial. One is influenced by the other, and it works both ways.

You are never without your personal psychology, and you are never totally separate from the world around you. Stay tuned to both aspects of your life while you are trying to lose weight.

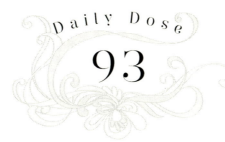

It takes the average smoker 8 to 10 times before she/he is able to quit successfully.

Can we take a lesson here? Is the habit of overeating any less hard to break than the habit of smoking?

No, it's just as hard; some might say it's even harder. You can quit smoking completely, but when it comes to overeating, you need to find a way to still eat, but not abuse it.

With smoking, tries at quitting involve falling off the wagon. This is typical. If a person quits for a year, though, she is very likely to stay off cigarettes forever.

If we take this to be true of bad eating habits as well, we can see at least that much time is required to change the habit.

Keep this in mind, and don't give up, even if you've failed before. Remember the "8 to 10 times" rule, and be encouraged to keep at it.

I am so great in a crisis. I can make order out of chaos and help everyone think clearly about what to do and how to handle things. I'm known for this. I rise to the occasion, don't lose my cool, never fall apart (until maybe after the crisis has passed). I amaze myself, and everyone around me.

I can even stick to a diet in the middle of a crisis. I figure out a way.

What I can't do very well is the everyday, the usual. That's when I have the most diet trouble—the day in, day-out part of staying on a diet. That's what's hard for me. It may sound crazy, but it's true.

Any thoughts?

Here's one. You seem to know in your mind and body and soul how to flip into crisis mode. You're all prepared with various strategies, and you don't need time to even think about it. It's like you're trained in this, and it works on the spot for you. You're a highly skilled crisis-negotiator.

OK, so what if you become skilled just like that in dealing with the everyday matters that tend to throw you off your diet? You could devise a plan to use on the spot when you are faced with any of the most diet-unfriendly situations, like maybe

You're exhausted

You're lonely

You're bored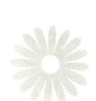

You're overworked

You have an argument with someone

The scale didn't move down enough

You have a cold

There's a chocolate cake in the house

You go out to dinner

Someone hurts your feelings

You're worried about your kid

These are the everyday kinds of things that can be so hard to reconcile with a diet.

Make a plan—details and all—for what you will do when these inevitable things come up. Have it ready. Try it out. Practice it. You'll soon be able to rise to these everyday occasions. The same way you became a great crisis-negotiator, you can become an expert, everyday negotiator.

Daily Dose

95

Cheating on your diet does not mean diet failure. Everyone does it at one point or another along the way. You most likely can't avoid it completely. What you can do is lessen the number of times you cheat, keep it to a minimum. The more you can stay on your diet, the more weight you'll lose.

An effective way to stall a cheat in its tracks is to stop and think. This is possibly the most powerful weight-loss technique you'll find. It takes some questioning, some considering, before you go ahead and plunge into those cookies and chips. Challenge yourself. See how flexible you can be. You don't need to do what you've always done. You can use your powers of thinking before you go ahead and cheat, thus avoiding self-recriminations and a reversal of your weight-loss progress.

Here is a checklist of questions that will steer you to the right kind of thinking. Use this list the next time you feel like cheating on your diet, before you actually do it. You can still cheat if you want to—that's always up to you. But once you answer these questions, even if you go ahead and cheat, it will be more of a real choice, and not just an automatic reflex.

Here is the Dieter's Cheating Checklist:

Am I still committed to losing weight?

What will the benefits to my life be when I reach my weight-loss goal?

Do I believe in my ability to stick to dieting?

If not, why not?

What are the strengths I possess that can help me stick to my diet right now?

Am I feeling very stressed out?

If so, can I handle the stress in some other way?

Am I tired?

If so, can I take some time out to rest?

Am I feeling overwhelmed?

If so, can I put off taking care of a few things until I feel more capable?

If I break my diet at this moment, will I feel better or worse?

If I cheat on my diet now, will I be able to get back on it?

Am I afraid to lose the weight?

If so, what am I afraid of?

What do I truly need right now?

Will eating off my diet plan give me what I need right now?

If not, how can I get what I need?

What would the people close to me think of me if I cheat now?

What will I think of myself if I cheat now?

If you have a problem with food and weight, you've probably trained yourself to turn to food at certain times. By now, it's probably an automatic response. You can use this checklist to retrain yourself. It can help make your dream of losing the weight once and for all come true.

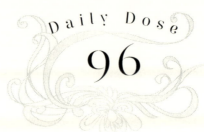

The morning after a big diet-busting meal, the
question is, how do you feel

about yourself

about the prospect of losing weight

about going back on the diet

about the future of this diet

about your ability to lose weight

Think about these questions next time you have a diet
power-failure. Because the trick is knowing it's not the
cheat itself that causes you to have the diet problem. It's
your reaction to a cheat that counts most.

Can you pick yourself up after a cheat, dust yourself off,
and keep at it? If so, you're on track for success.

What does not being able to stick to a diet reveal about you?

Maybe things like:

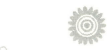

You hate to change

You are rebellious

You tend to get hopeless

You are not a good planner

You have trouble asking for help

You are afraid to lose the weight

You don't handle negative emotions well

You don't handle positive emotions well

You don't express your own needs enough

You are too self-critical

You give up on things too soon

You can't accept that you make mistakes

Diet, live, and learn.

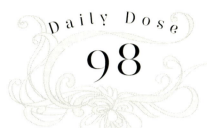

Cry if you want to. I can't cry over this any more.

So what will you do? Try to love being fat?

No, never. I need to get smart about it. About doing something about it.

So what's the answer?

I don't know. But I'm going to find one that works—for me, that is.

Good idea. Not possible.

You're so skeptical.

Shouldn't I be? How many times have we tried? Where are we now? Right back where we started.

My first parameter is that I will do something different this time—whatever it is, it will be something I've never even tried before.

I like the sound of that.

I need insight. I need to know what's been going wrong so I can figure out how to do it right.

I know. I can't even keep track of all the diet noise out there. It's overwhelming, and in the end it does me no good.

Me too. I think I need to reorganize my thinking and make it simpler. I guess what I mean is, I'll start with the problem itself. I need to state it more simply.

Like?

I don't know. But first of all I'll say something other than 'I've got to lose 30 pounds'. That's what I've said every time, and it's gotten me nowhere.

So?

Well this time I think I'll say, 'I've got to figure out why I can't stay on any diet for more than two weeks'.

Interesting.

In other words, the problem isn't so huge like losing 30 pounds. The problem is, why do I screw up after only two weeks every time I go on a diet?

That is fascinating, and reasonable. I think you can do that. I definitely think you can.

It seems like not such a big mountain to climb, know what I mean?

I do.

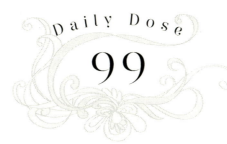

The littlest things can throw you.

Someone criticizes you in passing

You have a bad night's sleep

Someone disappoints you

You have one cheat

You look in the mirror and feel hopeless

You don't lose any weight at all one week

You have a very, very busy day

You get a cold

Little things can work against you while you're not looking.

Paying attention to small things can make a BIG difference.

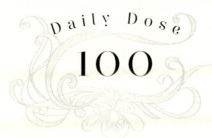

So, can you remember what you were thinking right before you ate the donuts?

Yes. It was like, if I don't eat these, I'll die.

Then after you ate them, did you feel better?

Yes, I did. It was a feeling of victory.

Can you say any more about how you were feeling before you ate the donuts?

Let's see. Well, I was tired. Exhausted, actually. And my daughter had to be driven to soccer practice, but I also needed to go to the store to get stuff for dinner. Then my husband called to say he'd be late.

Ah.

So I ate the donuts.

It sounds like you needed some sustenance to face all the things you had to do, even though you were tired.

I think so.

Do you remember how you felt after eating the donuts?

Yes. After the second one, I was feeling stuffed and uncomfortable.

So you needed something to eat, but already by the second donut you were feeling uncomfortable.

Yes.

It sounds like eating the donuts was a way of restoring yourself, but maybe you went too far by having so many.

And maybe part of it was I was angry at my husband for being late again. I desperately need help at the end of the day.

Do you think we could find a way for you to sustain yourself and express your anger without overdoing it in the food department?

Yeah. That would be good. Those three donuts made me feel stuffed, lazy, and more tired.

Let's see if we can think together about what you might do in this type of situation that would make you feel better, not worse.

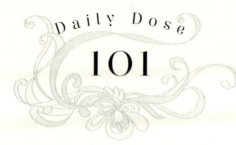

Dieting means restricting yourself.

So no matter what diet you choose to go on, there will be certain "no's"—certain things, or amounts, that you won't be able to eat.

You'll be saying "no" to yourself about these certain things if you're taking your diet seriously.

But let's consider the "yes" factor in dieting. Let's see what you'll be saying "yes" to by sticking with it . . .

I deserve to feel good.

I deserve to look good.

I am doing something important for myself.

I can learn to pursue long-term goals.

I can be a strong person.

I can think about what I want for myself.

I can be a little selfish sometimes.

I can put myself first when I need to.

I can think about my real needs.

I can work hard toward a goal.

I can start to feel good about myself.

Yes!

So what are a few "no's" compared to these great big "yes"
items?

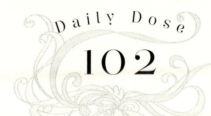

C an your diet still stick in these situations?

You're on a diet and your best friend makes a lavish surprise party for you, cake and all.

Chance of diet working   It probably won't. Just splurge, but STOP the splurge as soon as the party's over.

You're on a diet and you have a big fight with your husband over the household budget.

Chance of diet working   It's risky, but be determined to work out your money tensions without turning to food. Eating never fixes a financial problem.

You've dieted all week, but the scale hasn't budged.

Chance of diet working   Hold on here. It's a critical juncture. You need to understand that your body won't necessarily register a drop in pounds in direct relation to a good dieting week. Try sticking to your weight-loss diet faithfully for two more weeks—no weighing yourself. Then get on the scale. Give your body a chance to come through for you in it's own time.

No one is home and you get a great big urge to eat the tub of Dulce de Leche ice cream in the freezer.

Chance of diet working   Good chance, as long as you can ride out the wave of your urge. An urge has a time limit, and it runs it's course. If you can ride it out, it will lessen and dissipate, and then disappear. What a good feeling to get through the urge without giving in.

You're exhausted, and you have no willpower left.

Chance of diet working   Excellent. What you need to do is rest, and replenish your tired self. Give yourself what you actually need, and then you'll be able to stay on course.

A significant factor in being able to accomplish personal change is having helping relationships. You need to ask for support.

For some women, this is hard. Some don't feel they deserve help. Some don't want to appear too needy. Some think they should maintain a superwoman image, and let nothing spoil it.

Research shows that involving people close to you in something important you are trying to do actually helps you do it.

You use a diet to lose weight, right? But along with the diet's weight-loss function, you get other perks.

You can actually use the diet as a means for personal growth. If you work it right, a diet plan can expand your horizons by giving you more self-knowledge, better coping skills, and new strengths.

When you go on a diet, you are certainly changing the way you eat. But you are doing more than that. If you overeat, and you try to stop doing it, there will be the inevitable conflict between your habit of overeating and sticking to your diet. In order to settle this conflict in favor of sticking to the diet, you will need to face certain things about yourself. And if you are to lose the weight for good, you'll need to permanently change these things about yourself. And that's no easy matter.

Losing weight can yield personal triumphs beyond just pounds lost. It can be the journey of a lifetime.

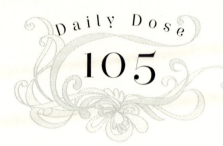

Daily Dose

105

HEAD: Now don't you dare eat that, you're on a diet.

HEART: I feel like a great big empty whole.

HEAD: You've already eaten your allotted calories, so don't be a pig.

HEART: I want to fill myself up to the top.

HEAD: Good things come to those who wait.

HEART: I need something NOW.

HEAD: See that woman? She looks good because she watches what she eats.

HEART: I hate anyone who's thin.

HEAD: Don't be a failure again.

HEART: I think I'm longing to be loved.

HEAD: Where's your willpower, woman?

HEART: Do you think I'll find enough love when I get to the bottom of this box of cookies?

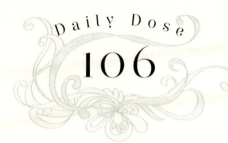

Sometimes people have ideas about themselves that aren't really true:

I simply must overeat

I have no willpower

I'm starving every minute of the day

I must lose fifty pounds

I need to have sweets every day

I could never give up cookies

I can't stick to a diet when I go out to eat

I'll never be able to lose the weight

I can't control my overeating

I must lose five pounds this week

I can't stand depriving myself of any food

I'm so fat it doesn't matter any more

Do you think of any of these things? If so, take the thoughts and do some "counterthinking". See if you can substitute truer thoughts.

Thought: I must overeat.

Better thought: I tend to overeat, but I think I can learn how not to.

or

Thought: I must lose five pounds this week.

Better thought: I'll stick to my diet this week, and I'm sure to starting losing weight.

or

Thought: I can't stand depriving myself of any food.

Better thought: When I am dieting, I tend to feel deprived, so I need to find ways of feeling fulfilled without using food.

What you tell yourself makes all the difference.

Let's say you've set your weight-loss goal. That's a start—a good start.

But in order for a goal to be effective, you need feedback as you go: It's essential. If you can't see how you are doing along the way, then you have no chance to make adjustments to the process.

You need to see where you are periodically in relation to the goal you've set. That way, you can see if you need to change anything about what you are doing. You may even find you are right on target, and then you can keep doing just what you are doing. If you are below target, or too much off the path, then you can try a new strategy, or modify the strategies you're using.

When the goal is losing weight, there are several ways to check progress. Keep an eye on:

How you feel

Your attitude

Changes in your eating behavior

How you look to yourself

How you are handling obstacles

How you are dealing with cheats

How your emotional life is going

Keep track. As you go, tweak things here and there, fix mistakes, capitalize on what works—all this enhances the probability of success.

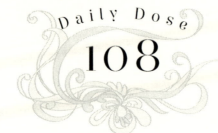

Did you know that making it public can make commitment to a weight-loss plan of action stronger?

You don't need to take out an ad in the newspaper. All you need to do is tell someone.

If you have decided to go on a diet, tell at least one person.

When you verbalize your weight-loss intentions to someone else, it strengthens your commitment. Not only that, by telling a trusted person you are setting up a support system. Since there is someone close to you who knows what you are trying to do, that's the very person you can go to for help when you need it.

Don't keep the diet a big secret. Your doubts about your abilities, your fears of failure, your tendency to quit when the going gets rough, all these things and more can be worked out with help.

Telling somebody outside of yourself about your decision to lose weight signals that you really mean to do it.

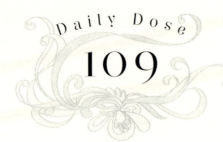

Daily Dose

109

Do you have a rigid pattern of behavior that you can't get out of?

Try stepping away from it. But do it gradually.

For example, let's say you're dying to reach a healthy weight. But your habit of dieting all day and stuffing it down at night is in your way.

Let's imagine how you can opt out of this self-defeating pattern.

Week 1

> Diet as usual during the days. When the times comes at night where you usually go off your diet, go off as usual, with one minor change: limit your falling-off to a half hour per night.

Week 2

> Diet as usual during the days. When your self-defeating habit comes into play at night, keep to

your limit of a nightly half hour falling-off, and add another slight change: pick one and only one non-diet food to eat.

Week 3

Once again, diet as usual during the day. Keep to the rule of weeks 1 & 2 with one minor change: limit your dieting holiday to only 15 minutes per night.

You see how it goes. These smaller, incremental steps serve as a guiding hand and help you let go of a behavior gradually.

Losing weight and becoming a smaller size is a way of re-inventing yourself. A gradual movement toward this new you will be much easier to achieve. The bad habit that was constantly stopping you from achieving weight loss, the self-defeating habit you thought you couldn't get away from, the habit you hated, will loosen its grip on you little by little, and finally die out.

Y ou're on a diet. You've committed yourself. Then you have a cheating episode. Do you attribute this instance of falling off your diet to your basic lack of willpower or a weakness in your character? Blaming such a lapse on fixed internal causes such as these can be problematic. It leads to a decreased sense of your own competence. Attributing a momentary failure to a rigid and unyielding negative personality characteristic makes you much more vulnerable to giving up.

Try this out. The next time you slip, instead of attributing the cause of your slip to internal "self" factors, turn your attention to the situational factors.

Take a careful look at the situation you were in when you slipped. Pay attention to the details. Where were you? Who were you with? What was going on around you? What was the occasion? What time of day was it? Try to consider this a specific, circumscribed situation that you couldn't cope with so well. This way, you open up a world of possibilities. For example, you can see that with more practice in situations like this, you'd be able to change your reaction. Or you could try to keep yourself away from such a situation. Or you could anticipate a situation like this and prepare for it.

Thinking like this leads to a greatly increased sense of self-efficacy—the sense of yourself as being capable. This increased sense of self-efficacy is the very thing to prevent a lapse from becoming a total relapse.

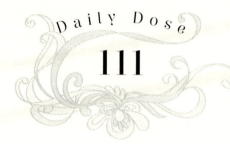

Daily Dose

111

When I go on a diet, within a week I meet with stiff resistance.

Who resists? Me.

So I'm sitting here trying to figure out why I resist my own desire to lose weight. It makes no sense.

I'm waiting and sitting, and nothing comes to me.

No one is telling me to lose weight. I'm telling myself. I really want to, and I've tried, believe me I've tried.

I tell myself this time will be different.

But it isn't.

Do you have any thoughts that might help me?

One thought is this: next time you go on a diet, and it's that dangerous first week, don't panic, don't fight too hard. In fact, let yourself do what you usually do, which is fall off. Your only job this time will be to notice what happens. Pay close attention to your thoughts and your feelings before, during, and after your diet smash-up. In other words, don't try so desperately to stay on. Instead, see what your stiff resistance is all about.

You are unlikely to be able to work through your resistance unless you can understand it. Once you can see more clearly how it works, why it works, what it does or doesn't do for you, that's when you get more power to overcome it. That's where the power and the know-how come from.

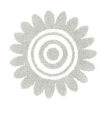

Y ou aren't born with it. It isn't innate. It is an acquired skill. Staying on your diet is something you can learn how to do.

How do you learn how? Well, the best way is to profit from your mistakes. That's the best way to learn how to do anything.

Let's say you are on a diet and you slip. What do you do now? This is the critical juncture. This is the part that separates the girls from the women. The moment to be reckoned with is right AFTER you have a diet lapse.

Always remember: our mistakes teach us the most. Mistakes are our mentors. Mistakes are our friends. Mistakes are our best dieting supports, if we know how to use them.

Take the last diet you went on. Can you recall a "falling off"? What did you do after? And here's the most important thing—what could you have done to turn the lapse into a tool for progress? Make a retro plan and imagine if you had done that. Would you and your diet have had a different outcome? Now take this very special dieting strategy with you into your next diet.

Staying on a diet is indeed something you can learn how to do. Look for those mistakes and use them to your advantage.

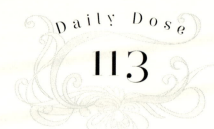

What do researchers find when they study dieters who go on different diet plans?

NO DIET WILL WORK UNLESS YOU CAN STICK TO IT.

Most people can't stick to a diet plan very well, even the best diet, the healthiest diet plan, the trendiest, the newest, the quickest, the one with the most protein, the one with the lowest fat, or even the most balanced plan there is. People just plain have trouble sticking to a diet, no matter what one chooses.

So here's the best advice. Make a non-food plan to go along with your diet. Map out an "obstacle course". What do you see yourself running up against when you go on your next diet? What are the obstacles?

For example:

> temptations, holidays, fatigue, busy schedule, sadness, anger, disappointment, kids, parents,

friends, weekends, emergencies, lack of support, hopelessness, the aftermath of cheating, hunger, emotional emptiness, impatience

You can think beforehand about what always pops up to derail your diet. Then make a plan. What will you do when these things present themselves?

This non-food plan is more important than the diet you choose.

IT'S NEVER, NEVER JUST ABOUT THE FOOD.

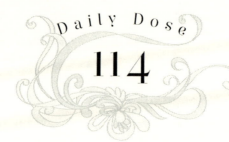

Daily Dose

114

Dear Eating Problem (EP) . . .

What do you know about me?

EP: A lot.

me: Whisper to me. Tell me my secrets.

EP: Are you sure you want to know?

me: No.

EP: Well then, let's just continue as we are.

me: No good.

EP: Why not? It's been working OK so far.

me: I'm not so sure. You come off without a hitch. You work really well. You're in great shape. I'm not.

EP: Better not rock the boat.

me: Why not?

EP: Because, then you might get nervous.

me: Maybe I can take it.

EP: Maybe, maybe not.

me: So what's the worst that can happen?

EP: You'll feel terrible.

me: I feel terrible now.

EP: You're asking me to let you go, aren't you?

me: I am.

EP: But we've been together for so long. What will you do without me?

me: I don't know, but it's time I find out.

EP: OK then. Til we meet again.

me: No. Goodbye.

Losing weight is about more than you think.

Losing weight is like any other life journey. There are peaks and valleys, success and failures, hopes and disappointments.

If you keep a sense of adventure as you go through the journey, you will find it's a learning experience that goes way beyond figuring out how to lose weight. It teaches you about the best and worst parts of yourself. It teaches you about courage and fear. It teaches you about stamina. It teaches you how to stretch your capabilities, and how to overcome obstacles. It teaches you about self-esteem, pride, needs, feelings, defenses, and the human art of making mistakes.

The successful weight-loss journey makes you lighter, but it's not to be taken lightly.

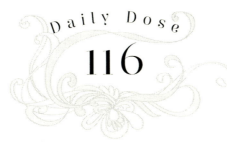

Are you on a diet?

Are you planning to go on a diet?

Grab a notebook, or start a "diet journal" file on your computer. Every day, make notes about at least one of the following:

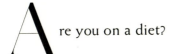

The effort it's taking

Sharpening your skills

Making progress

Enjoyable parts

Difficult parts

What you are discovering

Your expectations

Your feelings of accomplishment

Communicate with yourself as you go. It works wonders to stay in touch with what you are going through.

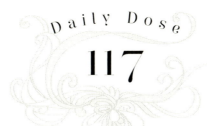

If you have dieted and lost weight in the past, and then gone back to your old ways, you have a lot of strength.

Does that sound counterintuitive? It's not. If you think about it, you went ahead and took action. Lots of people don't do that. They think about dieting, they want to, they feel they should, but thinking is all they do.

But if you are a relapser, you have that experience of taking action. OK, so you didn't follow through the whole way. But you started; that's big. And you can start again. Not only that, but you can take that try, or as many times as you've tried before, and use what you learned as a guide.

And you can do much better this time, especially if you can answer yes to the following questions:

> Do you understand the major causes of your past dieting failure(s)?

Can you make a better plan to deal with these causes next time?

Can you try with all your might to go back on your diet and not give up after you have a momentary lapse?

Can you make this weight-loss challenge an absolute priority in your life this time?

Take strength and courage from the fact that you had the strength to try before . . . and try again.

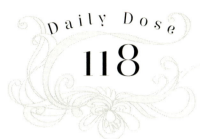

Daily Dose

118

I t enhances your dieting chances to know what dances
in your head!

There are thoughts and ideas that trigger problem
behaviors like overeating. The thoughts may come so
under your radar that you aren't aware you're having them.

You can do something about this. You can increase your
awareness of what goes on in your head preceding an
instance of breaking your diet.

You may find that overeating isn't even something you
enjoy. It might serve a totally different purpose. It might
act as an anti-anxiety medication. It might act as an anger
reducer. It might be an act of rebelliousness.

Then there is the consequence of your behavior. What are
your thoughts after you indulge? Do you rationalize? Do
you try to justify what you've done? Do you have deep
regrets? Do you wish you hadn't done it?

See if you can catch hold of what you are thinking before
you eat too much, and what you are thinking after. This
is a kind of consciousness-raising technique that helps
you move away from unwanted behavior, toward self-
enhancing behavior.

Even though there may be reasons why you know you should lose weight, that is only a first step. It is an important step to acknowledge the need to do it, but it's not enough in and of itself.

The next step in the process of losing weight is commitment. Commitment means that you are basically ready to move the task of losing weight to the top of your agenda.

This requires that you be willing to put a good deal of emphasis on losing weight. It means being able to dedicate time and energy to the cause.

Even when you realize that you want to lose weight, if you are not in the frame of mind to put forth the effort it will take, you will undermine your efforts.

Go ahead and make the decision to lose weight. Then support that decision by committing yourself to making it a central task of your life, for whatever time it takes.

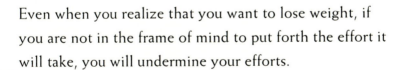

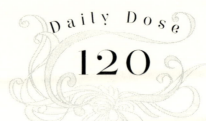

Are you at a weight you hate?

Want to build your dieting muscle?

Exercise your power of thinking.

In order to lose weight, don't lose your mind, use it!

Think about

> When you overeat
>
> Why you overeat
>
> How you feel before you overeat
>
> How you feel after you overeat
>
> What you might do instead of overeating
>
> How you would feel if you lose the weight
>
> How you will feel if you don't

It's mind/body, always. The connection is there; it is undeniable.

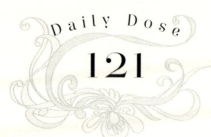

If you can't ever seem to stick to a diet, no doubt you have a system in place. The trouble is, it's your weight *maintaining* system.

Can you disrupt this system? That's exactly your job if you want to solve the sticking-to-it problem. The idea is to disturb the status quo by doing something different.

Suppose whenever you go to a restaurant, the food on the menu sounds so good that your dieting goes right out the window. You don't want to miss anything; you overeat; you go home feeling terribly disappointed in yourself.

Now let's suppose someone said to you, "Can you think of any exception to this? Can you think of any time at all when you did not do this?" Let's say you do recall a time when you were able to hold on. You were able to stick to your dieting resolve, even though you were at a restaurant. Perhaps you did it by reminding yourself how important losing the weight was to you. This instance would be a real exception to the rule, and remembering it can show you that you are capable of doing something different. Now you would be acknowledging that you have it within you to act in a more constructive way.

Try it out. Can you think of an anti-dieting habit that you have firmly in place? Think of one exception to your habit, a time when you broke your own rule. Let yourself see that you are capable of doing something out of your ordinary, something more in your best interest, something that keeps you on track. And if you could do it once, why can't you do it again? And then again.

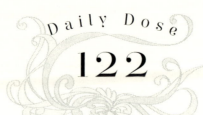

Daily Dose

122

Dieters beware!

There are three types of situations to be particularly mindful of. These are the situations most likely to pull you off your food plan, and send you back to your old eating habits.

You are experiencing a negative mood or negative emotions.

You are involved in interpersonal conflict with either family or friends.

You are facing stressful life conditions such as financial difficulties, loss of job, a child leaving home, etc.

These situations put you at significant risk for dieting failure. Be aware.

C an your genes tell you what diet to go on?

There's a study from Stanford University that found if you take a test to see how you burn and store calories based on your individual genetic makeup, it will help you find the diet that matches you best. It seems that finally, you'll know whether to go on a low-carb or a low-fat food plan.

Some weight-loss experts are skeptical of this study. But Mindy Dopler Nelson, a nutritional biologist at Stanford who conducted the study, reports that women on diets matched to their genes lose more weight than women on random diets.

This certainly sounds like an exciting approach for women who want to lose weight. After all, genetic research is now leading to all kinds of new ideas and treatments for illnesses and lifestyle issues.

Here's what Dr. Robert Eckel, former president of

The American Heart Association says with regard to the new study: STICKING WITH A DIET IS MORE IMPORTANT THAN WHAT DIET YOU CHOOSE.

You can be tested and tested until a diet is found that matches your physical makeup and your metabolism perfectly. But even the most perfect match-up won't ensure that you will be able to stay on that diet.

Sticking to it is a very sticky matter. The diet counts, yes, but the crucial issue is whether or not you can stay with that diet. Because if you can't, what good is any diet?

Let's say this genetic testing is valid, and you go ahead to have it. Suppose it concludes that you just don't metabolize carbohydrates well. You are convinced. You even know from past experience this is true. Let's say you even tried a low-carb diet before and it seemed to work well. So how come you're not thin?

Well, either you couldn't stick with it, or after the diet you went back to your old ways and gained it back. These are the 2 MOST IMPORTANT factors in weight-loss failure. These are the issues that must be addressed, even if you go on the most perfect diet of all.

Daily Dose

124

Here's a good way to stay the course when you're on a diet: Be kind to yourself. Empathy and understanding facilitate change.

Accept your ambivalence. You won't be totally committed every minute of every day. When those other thoughts come—"I don't want to be on a diet"—respect them as part of who you are.

Think of your goals and values. When you come up against a difficult time during your diet, ask yourself: What is my goal here? What can I do now to help me get there? What would keep me from getting there now?

Remember about your personal strengths. Believing in your ability to persevere is key. Strengthen your confidence from time to time by reminding yourself of your abilities. Recall other times in your life when your personal strengths helped you stick to a task that was important to you.

Don't use a cheat to berate yourself. Instead, use every mistake as a tool. Almost everyone cheats on a diet at some time or other. Go easy on your imperfect, perfectly human self.

You can definitely develop the art of *sticking to it*. It requires a kind, gentle, appreciative attitude toward yourself, above all.

Once you find yourself in cheating mode, it can be very hard to get out of it. One cheat leads to the next, and so on. Grabbing onto the diet again can get more difficult with each cheat.

The way to handle a cheat is to not let it evolve into a continuing spiral of off-the-diet eating.

If you are on a diet, and you've been indulging in cheat after cheat, don't give up! You can snap out of it.

Here is a damage-control technique for getting back on the diet wagon, even if you've been falling off like crazy:

PLAN your cheats from now on. Decide what day, how long it will last, and even what you will eat. Planned cheating can really help put you back in control.

Don't just let it slide, because then you run the risk of giving up altogether. Try this strategy. It is very good for getting you back into diet-success mode.

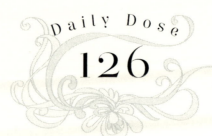

Here's a funny question: What do you expect from yourself?

For example, when you go on a diet, do you actually expect yourself to be successful? Or, do you expect yourself to fail? Think about it.

This may seem like an inconsequential question, but really it's a big one. Because what you expect yourself to do can greatly influence what you actually do.

Try to answer this question, and be honest. Even if the answer is that you expect yourself to be a diet failure, you can figure out how you can change your expectations. What would actually make you feel like you can do it?

Expecting failure makes you fail; expecting success makes you succeed.

When you are trying to lose weight, the main players are WILLPOWER and WON'T POWER. They share the spotlight. And they don't have a thing to do with food.

> I WILL try to stay in touch with my moods and my feelings
> I WON'T try to feel better by overeating
>
> I WILL remember that self-change is a process
> I WON'T try to rush it
>
> I WILL carve out time for rest and relaxation
> I WON'T take on too many other obligations right now
>
> I WILL treat myself with respect and appreciation
> I WON'T be too self-critical

I WILL get help and/or support from a professional or
    someone close to me
I WON'T attempt this journey all by myself

I WILL accept and learn from my mistakes
I WON'T give up on myself

I WILL work on the non-food issues
I WON'T let myself forget that it's never, never just
    about the food

True Willpower and Won't-power produce the results you
are looking for.

Y ou can stick to it when it's easy; you can stick to it when it's not.

You can stick to it by thinking; you can stick to it by feeling.

You can stick to it by looking forward; you can stick to it by looking back.

You can stick to it by falling; you can stick to it by getting back up.

You can stick to it with answers; you can stick to it with questions.

You can stick to it at home; you can stick to it on the fly.

You can stick to it at first; you can stick to it as you go.

You can stick to it when it's raining; you can stick to it in snowstorms.

You can stick to it like glue; you can stick to it like post-its.

You can stick to it with food; you can stick to it with much more than food.

Also by the authors

Breaking Up With Food

Maria's Last Diet

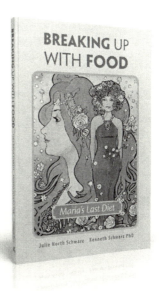

"When Maria came into a room she was there, no doubt. She generated warmth, excitement, and interest. Her voice was distinctively clear and friendly. In a social setting, she was "on", making sure no one could get through the surface to break her apart into smaller pieces, to melt her down into the atoms of self-doubt she was made of."

Welcome to the world of Maria. She is an "everywoman", yet as unique and quirky a person as you'd ever want to meet. In her own way, Maria struggled mightily against a weight problem for many years before she was able to solve it. This is an inside peek, for weight loss—permanent weight loss—always comes from the inside out. Its path is strewn with secrets revealed, and that is what makes it a deep and uplifting adventure.

The story of Maria's last diet is a story of suspense, mystery, daring, and victory. This book isn't just about Maria. It's fiction, but there is a real story behind it. It's Maria; it's you; it's any woman who has trouble dieting; it's for those who can't stay on a diet, for those who can stay on but at some point gain it all back; it's for those who keep trying and failing, for those who keep dreaming about losing weight, and for those who have given up the dream.

This is a story about disappointment, failure, and heartbreak. This is a story of learning, accepting, knowing, hoping, and trying. This is a success story.

An interactive system for diet mastery

DietTuffy.com

a serious online game

. . . to get rid of obstacles to weight loss . . .

from **DietInReview.com**

> "Diet Tuffy is meant to "toughen" you up so that you are
> equipped with the right tools and plans to make your
> next diet a success."

> "Diet Tuffy might be just the solution for you to finally
> overcome your diet challenges and lose the weight for
> good."

No doubt you have found that dieting is hard. Why? Because like
so many other women, you always have to fight against certain
problems that pop up when you diet. In order to diet successfully,
you need to solve problems like:

- low motivation

- vulnerability to temptations

- emotional eating

- feeling deprived

- negative thinking

- hard to break habits

- low self-confidence

Diet Tuffy

is the dieter's online problem solver.

Come and take the 5 seriously fun and confidence-building steps.

- **First:** You will zero in on a significant problem you have as a dieter. You can use our universal list of dieting problems to help you specify a problem, or you can put it in your own words.

- **Next:** You will come up with a brand new solution to your problem.

- **Then:** You will see how to make an ingenious plan to put your new solution right into action.

- **After that:** You will mentally film your plan to see where it gets hung up.

- **And last:** You will fine tune your plan to make doubly sure it works.

At the end of your Diet Tuffy interactive experience, you will have a solid plan in hand to overcome your dieting problem.

Once you have used Diet Tuffy to solve a problem, it is yours to come back to (free of charge) as many times as you like . . . to solve any other dieting problems you may have.

Solving your anti-diet problems is exactly how to make your diet work next time.

Check it out at

DietTuffy.com

About the Authors

Kenneth Schwarz PhD is a psychologist and psychoanalyst practicing in Connecticut, where he is an allied health staff member at Sharon Hospital. Julie North Schwarz is a writer in the field of women's weight issues. Together they are the driving force behind *MariasLastDiet.com*, a website for women that is all about the psychological side of dieting and weight loss. Their first novel, *Breaking Up With Food: Maria's Last Diet*, was published in 2010 by Symmetry Press.

The Schwarzes make their home in the northwest corner of Connecticut, USA., where they have lots of get-togethers with Paul, Caro, Theo, Joanna, Chris, Ellie, and Julian.

Breinigsville, PA USA
11 November 2010
249100BV00001B/18/P